OUSSHA SHLAIMOUN

PURE
CURE

THE WHOLE FAMILY GUIDE
TO WHOLE LIFE WELLNESS

Pure Cure: A Family Guide to Wellness
by Oussha Shlaimoun

Copyright © 2016 by Oussha Shlaimoun

ISBN: 978-1-944177-21-8 (p)
ISBN: 978-1-944177-22-5 (e)

Cover Design by Melody Hunter

Crescendo Publishing, LLC
300 Carlsbad Village Drive
Ste. 108A, #443
Carlsbad, California 92008-2999

1-877-575-8814
GetPublished@CrescendoPublishing.com

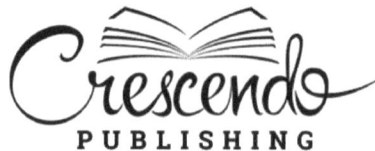

Crescendo
PUBLISHING

PURE CURE: A FAMILY GUIDE TO WELLNESS
Oussha Shlaimoun

ABOUT THE BOOK

Pure Cure, a family guide to wellness, is a handy reference tool for treating common ailments using natural means. It draws from my knowledge of homeopathy, of oils and flower essences, of super foods, herbs, and teas. Since we're all different, what works for one person may not work for another. Pure Cure is designed to complement conventional medicine, to guide the reader in choosing an alternative protocol that may be just right for them and since most natural remedies do not interact with prescription drugs, many can be used in conjunction with prescription drugs or alternatively as a last resort, when all else has failed.

I decided to write this book when, to my astonishment, I realized that most people aren't aware of the natural alternatives that exist and that prescription medication isn't the only option. Nature has provided us with an effective medicine cabinet that doesn't have many of the nasty side effects that prescription medications suffer from.

ABOUT HOMEOPATHY

Homeopathy is one of the oldest systems of medicine. Homeopathy Is practiced around the World by millions of people. The principle of homeopathy is "like cures like," so if your symptom is a rash, a homeopath would prescribe a remedy causing a rash. Homeopathy believes that disease causes symptoms, so if you want to get better, you need to cure the disease rather than the symptom. Homeopathy has thousands of remedies, most of which are highly diluted and act on a person's mental and emotional state.

USING THIS BOOK

This book is a guide to help you understand what natural protocols are available to you and although I tried to cover many common ailments, I've only scratched the surface in this book. This book is designed to steer you in the right direction, to try a new approach, and to look outside the confines of allopathic medicines. It is not intended to replace your physician's diagnosis, advice and protocol but to complement it.

Some conditions can be very dangerous and life threatening, so proper diagnosis and management is essential. Please be sure to consult a professional health practitioner, if you have any medical questions. You should also let your professional health practitioner know if you are taking any other protocols or natural remedies. The dosages and usages for each aliment vary from person to person, depending on the severity of the condition and condition of the patient. You are encouraged to discuss these recommendations and protocols with your holistic and health care practitioner before beginning any recommendation outlined in this book and always remember, what works for one person may not work for another. So it is important to try different options, to see what works best for you.

And please remember that I am not responsible for the decisions and health of anyone else but myself. I do not make any claims that any of these recommendations will work for you; instead, I share with you my knowledge of what works for me and my family.

I hope the information in this book helps you and should you have any non medical questions or comments, please don't hesitate to contact me via my website www. rightremedy.com.

| DEDICATION

This book is dedicated to my family—my husband and our two sons. They believed in me, supported me, and encouraged me to better myself and to better our lives. It is also dedicated to those who shared my journey, to those who taught me, and those who learnt from me. To my courageous mum who battled and defeated cancer, to my dad, my sister and to Mandy for their support, help and encouragement.

To those who aren't mentioned here (you know who you are), for their positiveness and their energy. You all played a vital role.

In this book I've included standard potencies for homeopathic remedies, e.g. Arnica 30c. Please remember that the potency I have listed is only a guideline and should be adjusted depending on your energy level. So the higher your energy, the higher the potency. However, Chronic illnesses (i.e. those you've had for a long time) should be treated with low potencies (6c) and Acute conditions (i.e. those that are relatively new) with high potencies (100c)

TABLE of CONTENTS

PURE CURE:
The Whole Family Guide to Whole Life Wellness

Oussha Shlaimoun

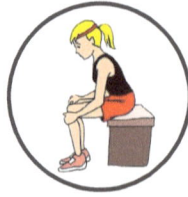

ACHING MUSCLES

Aching muscles are caused by a buildup of lactic acid in the muscle (e.g., following a hard training session or lifting heavy weights), dehydration, and a lack of the mineral calcium in your diet. But not all muscle aches are related to tension and physical activity. Some aches can be caused by infection, lupus, or even flu.

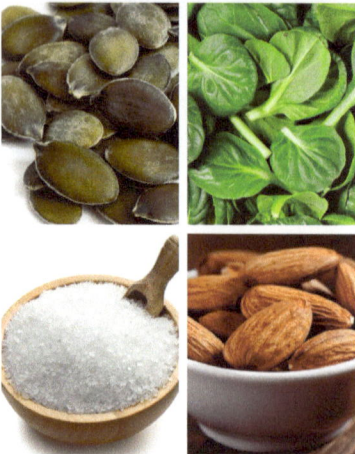

HOMEOPATHIC

One dose at intervals of 15-30 minutes for 2 doses

- Arnica 30c
- Rhus Toxicodendron 30c
- Ruta Graveolens 30c

ESSENTIAL OILS

- Peppermint (4 drops mixed with a carrier oil)
- Clove (4 drops mixed with a carrier oil)
- Lemon (4 drops mixed with a carrier oil)

VITAMINS

- Magnesium one tablet twice a day

FOODS

Most foods that contains magnesium, including;

- Pumpkin seeds
- Spinach
- Almonds
- Organic Blackstrap molasses (Sulfur-Free)

GENERAL

- Epsom salt (natural muscle relaxant that helps expel excess fluids from the tissues, reducing swelling) in bath
- Hot or cold ice pack (applied to muscle)

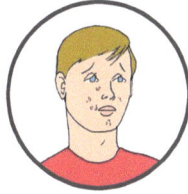

ACNE

Acne vulgaris is a chronic skin condition characterized by the outbreak of black-heads, whiteheads, pim-ples, redness, swelling, and greasy skin.

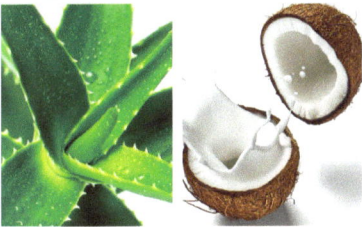

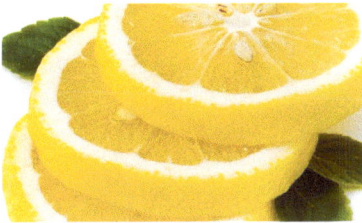

FOODS

- Whole foods and lean poultry
- Hormone-free meats and eggs, as acne is influenced by hormonal factors
- Soya, rice, or coconut milk
- Glass of water mixed with about two teaspoons of apple-cider vinegar
- Diet with special emphasis on fibrous and nutritious fruits, vegetables, nuts, seeds, and whole grains, especially the ones rich in vitamin A and vitamin E
- Aloe vera juice

LIFESTYLE

- Stress can increase levels of cortisol and worsen acne
- Applying a combination of three tablespoons of honey and one teaspoon of cinnamon powder to the affected area
- Honey can also be used along with egg whites to remove acne cysts naturally at home
- Mix equal parts of baking soda and water to form a paste. Preferably, add some sea salt as well and then apply this paste to the affected area.
- Rinse face with apple-cider vinegar.
- 1 Aspirin mask mixed with 2 tablespoon water or 1 tablespoon Aloe Vera
- Half tablespoon lemon applied on the pimple helps dry out pimples. Lemon can also be used with egg white to dry up pimples.
- For inflammation and acne scars apply turmeric ¾ tablespoon, together with half a tablespoon of honey and 1 tablespoon plain yogurt.

ACNE
continued

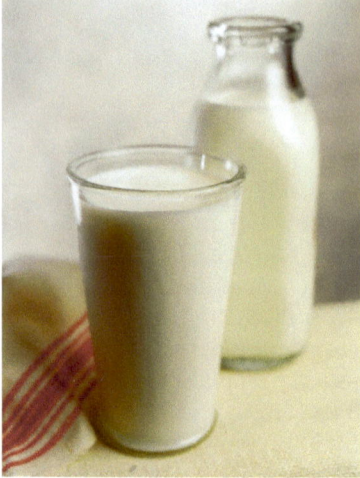

AVOID

- Junk and processed foods, such as white-flour products
- Cow's milk (aggravates acne in some patients)

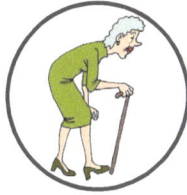

AGING

Aging is another name for the process of becoming older. As the body ages, it changes over time. The process of aging is not reversible and may make you feel tired, even drained. You may also notice wrinkles, painful joints, and age spots.

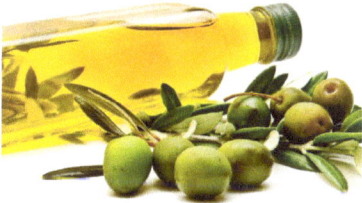

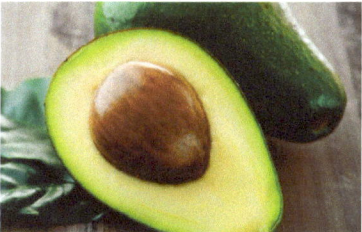

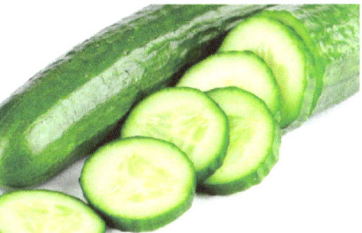

HOMEOPATHIC
- Avena-Sativa (increases life span) 30c

ESSENTIAL OILS
Use 2 drops of oil with 10ml coconut oil and apply on face
- Rose-hip seed (smooths out wrinkles)
- Carrot seed (rejuvenates skin)
- Apricot kernel (wrinkle-prevention oil)
- Coconut oil (delays sagging skin)

VITAMINS
- Vitamin C one a day
- Coenzyme one in the morning
- Vitamin E one a day
- Ashwangandha (slows aging process)

FOODS
- Alkaline water with fresh, organic lemon
- Papaya
- Avocados
- Cucumbers
- Organic orange juice
- Goji berries
- Organic carrots
- Organic lemons
- Goats Milk (applied to skin before sleep)
- Olive oil

TEAS
Drink 3X Daily
- White (fights effects of aging)
- Red rooibos (helps premature aging)
- Green tea (improves longevity)

9

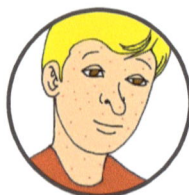

ALLERGIES

Allergies occur when your immune system reacts to foreign substances and produces antibodies. Some allergies are inherited from your family, and some develop as a result of touching something. An allergic reaction can be brought on by breathing in or eating an allergen. When an allergic reaction does occur, the body releases histamine into the bloodstream.

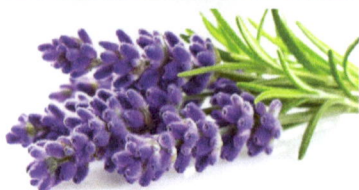

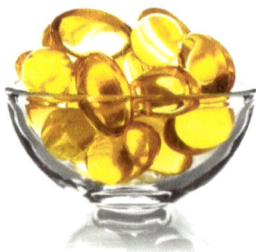

HOMEOPATHIC

- Arsenicum 6c 3 x daily depending on how you are feeling as soon as you feel better stop taking remedy (same with all homeopathic remedies especially during acute state)
- Histamine 30c
- Pollen 30c
- Allium Cepa all depends on what type of allergy you have so you would need to see a professional homeopath to know what to take on an acute level .
- Apis 30c
- Mixed Pollen 30c
- Phosphorus 30c
- Sabadilla 6c
- Psorinum 6c

ESSENTIAL OILS

- Lavender
- Eucalyptus (inhale steam)
- Almond (inserted with a Q-TIP inside nostrils; protects against pollen getting in)
- Half tablespoon lemon applied on the pimple helps dry out pimples. Lemon can also be used with egg white to dry up pimples.
- For inflammation and acne scars apply turmeric ¾ tablespoon, together with half a tablespoon of honey and 1 tablespoon plain yogurt.

ALLERGIES
continued

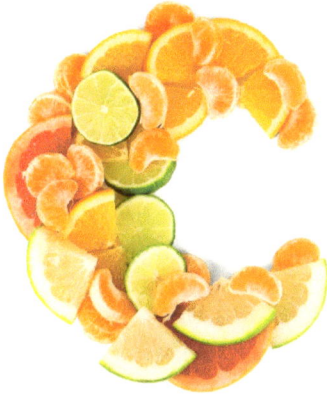

VITAMINS
- Vitamins C, D and E once a day
- Zinc

FOODS
- Bee pollen from your area

HERBS
- Butterbur
- Quercetin

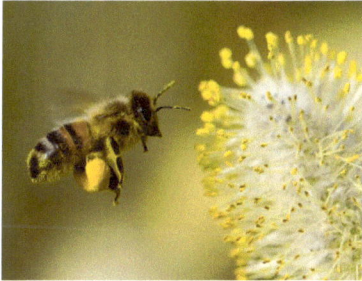

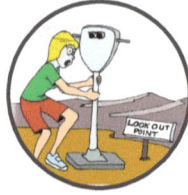

ALTITUDE SICKNESS

Altitude sickness (also known as acute mountain sickness) is the effect of low oxygen pressure at high altitude. It commonly occurs above 8,000 feet and can make a person feel like they are hungover.

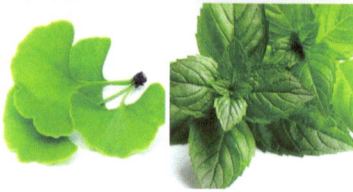

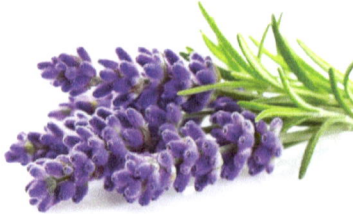

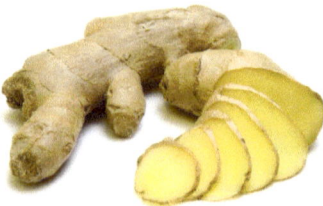

HOMEOPATHIC

- Kali Phos 30c
- Cocculus 6c take 3 x a day especially during acute state, depending on your symptom.
- Pulsatilla 6c
- Arsenicum Album 30c
  It is safe to take these remedies as frequently as every ten minutes but you should contact a qualified homeopath.

ESSENTIAL OILS

- Peppermint
- Lavender
- Ginger

VITAMINS

- Gingko
  (read instructions on the bottle)
- Ginger
- Arginine
- Selenium
- Vitamin C (recommended dosage is 2,000 to 3,000 milligrams per day)

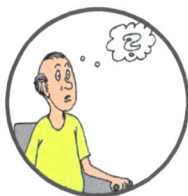

ALZHEIMER'S DISEASE

Alzheimer's disease is a progressive disease that destroys memory and other important mental functions. With no known cure and a terminal prognosis, Alzheimer's disease is associated with degeneration and death in brain cells, leading to a steady loss of both intellectual and social skills, loss of functional daily abilities, and, ultimately, premature death.

HOMEOPATHIC

- Baryta Carbonica 6c
- Nat Sulpuricum 6c
- Nux Vomica 30c

ESSENTIAL OILS

- Lavender
- Lemon Balm
- Peppermint (put one drop of essential oil on a tissue and inhale through the nose)
- Rosemary
- Bergamot
- Ginger

VITAMINS

- Ashwagandha take as recommended
- Evening primrose take one a day
- Garlic take one a day
- Ginseng take one twice a day
- Turmeric take one a day
- Vitamin E take one a day
- B12 take one a day

FOODS

- Walnuts
- Salmon
- Spinach
- Coffee
- Chocolate (dark)
- Blueberries
- Introduce more healthy fats to your diet (e.g. Avocado)

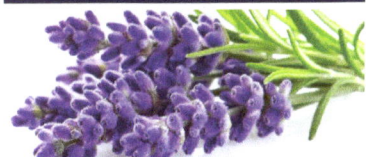

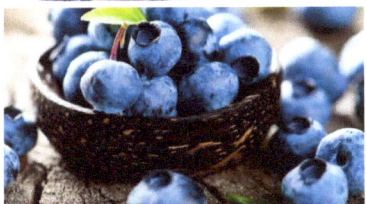

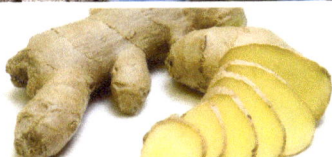

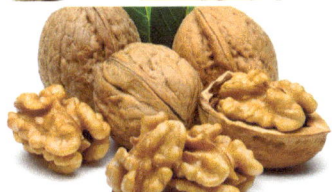

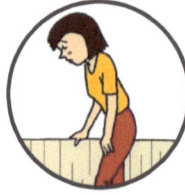

ANEMIA

Anemia is a decrease in red blood cells that can be caused by blood loss, or by not having enough B6, folic acid, B12, or copper in the system. Signs of anemia include feeling fatigued, dizziness, shortness of breath, paler skin color, and low blood pressure.

HOMEOPATHIC
- Ferrum Phos 30c once a day
- Pulsatilla 30c
- Nat Muriaticum 30c

ESSENTIAL OILS
- Lemon mixed with 50 ml almond carrier oil

FOODS
- Green, leafy vegetables
- Egg yolk
- Yogurts
- Beets
- Lentils
- Blackstrap molasses (contains vast amounts of iron)
- Clams
- Dried apricots
- Broccoli
- Healthy Fats (e.g. Avocado, olive oil, fish oil)

AVOID
- Coffee (decreases iron absorption)

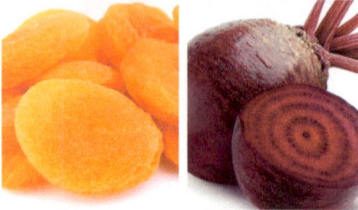

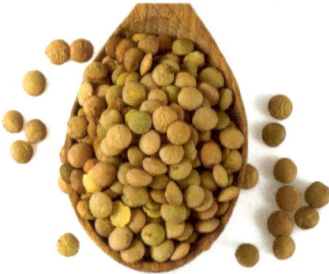

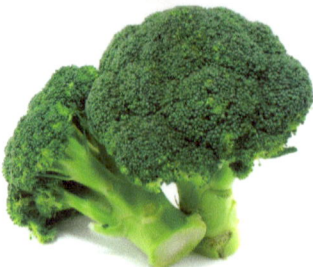

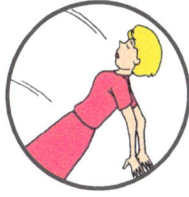

ANAPHYLACTIC SHOCK

Anaphylactic shock is an allergic reaction that may be triggered by certain kinds of insect bites, drugs, and/or food groups. It is important to keep your immune system healthy, especially your liver.

HOMEOPATHIC

- Arnica 6c
- Apis 30c
- Phosphorus 6c

ESSENTIAL OILS

Very important you check with your doctor before using any oils. 2 drops with carrier oil

- Lavender
- Peppermint
- Lemongrass

VITAMINS

Always refer to instructions on the bottle or contact a naturopathic doctor.

- Vitamin C
- Zinc
- Echinacea
- Ginkgo Biloba

FOODS

- Citrus fruits
- Apples
- Onions
- Parsley
- Sage

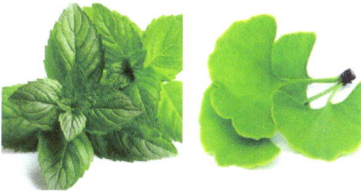

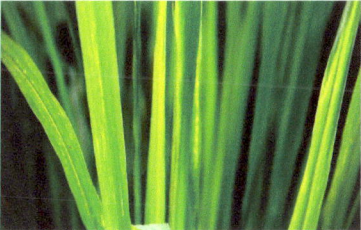

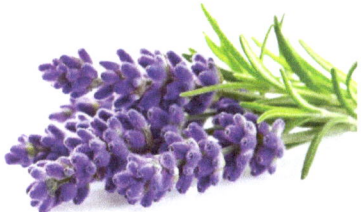

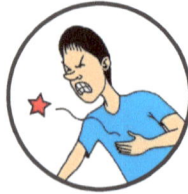

ANGINA

Angina occurs when the heart muscle does not get enough blood supply and oxygen. Symptoms of angina include pressure/squeezing sensation in the chest.

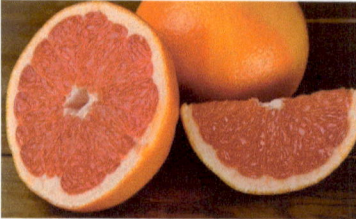

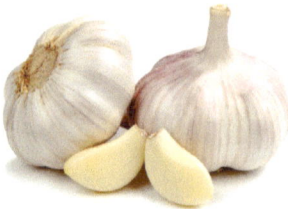

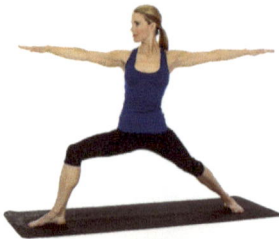

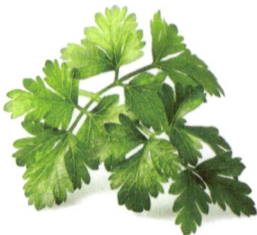

HOMEOPATHIC
- Amyl Nitrate 30c
- Crataegus 6x
- Glonoine 30c
- Spigelia 30c

VITAMINS
- L-Carnitine one a day
- Coenzyme Q10 one a day
- Vitamin A consult your doctor before taking
- Vitamin C one a day

FOODS
- Fish oils (e.g. Omega 3, 6 and 9)
- Garlic
- Parsley
- Grapefruit (tones up heart)
- Lemon

LIFESTYLE
- Hawthorn 10 drops in the evening
- Crataegus 10 drops in 8oz of water in the morning
- Yoga or other moderate exercise

AVOID
- Fatty foods (e.g. fried foods)
- Caffeine

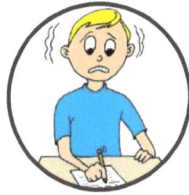

ANXIETY

Anxiety is an unpleasant state of inner turmoil, often accompanied by nervous behavior and feelings of dread over anticipated events known as the "fight or flight" response. Causes of anxiety include genetics, stress, brain chemistry, and psychological issues. Negative self-talk can also affect your anxiety levels, in addition to a lack of oxygen in high-altitude areas. Illness can also have an effect on your anxiety levels. Anxiety is a difficult emotion to cope with and can cause insecurity, irritability, and restlessness.

HOMEOPATHIC

- Aconite (first acute remedy on onset of anxiety attack)
- Gelsemium
- Arg-Nitricum
- Arsenicum Album
- Nat-Muriaticum

ESSENTIAL OILS

- Frankincense
- Lavender (helps nervous system)
- Ylang ylang

VITAMINS

- Kava take one in the morning and one in the evening
- Folic acid take one in the morning
- Vitamin B complex take one in the morning
- Valerian take one in the evening
- Magnesium take one morning and in the evening

HERBAL TEAS

- Chamomile drink 3 to 4 cups in a day

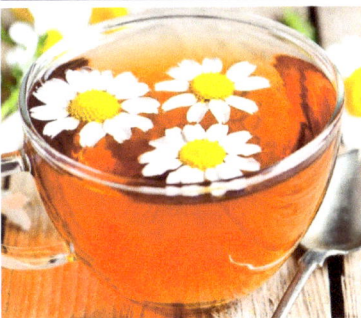

ANXIETY
continued

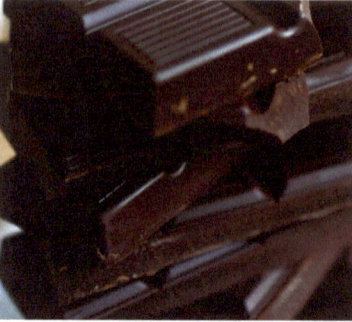

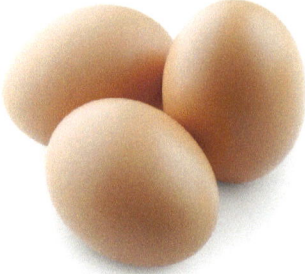

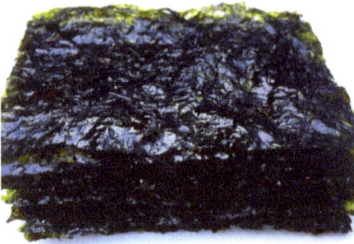

FOODS

- Turkey (has tryptophan)
- Bananas
- Chicken
- Sesame seeds
- Oats
- Peanut butter
- Seaweed (high content of magnesium)
- Blueberries
- Almonds (magnesium)
- Dark chocolate (helps with moods)
- Eggs (Vitamin B helps with nervous system)

LIFESTYLE

- Keeping hydrated
- Exercise helps burn away stress
- Breathing exercise (e.g., breathe in 4 times and breathe out 5 times)
- Cognitive behavioural therapy
- Meditation
- Yoga headstand positions (increases blood flow to the head)

AVOID

- Unrefined sugar
- Alcohol
- Fried foods

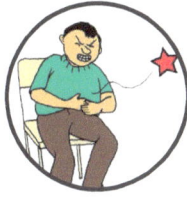

APPENDICITIS

The appendix is a small, finger-like intestine in the lower right side of the abdomen. Appendicitis is an inflammation of the appendix, usually caused by the obstruction of the appendiceal lumen. The obstruction leads to distention and inflammation.

HOMEOPATHIC

- Belladonna 30c
- Bryonia 30c
- Arsenicum 30c
- Rhus Ticodendron 30c

FOODS

- Cucumber juice
- Beets
- Ginger
- Wild yam

HERBS

Take up to 10 drops in 8oz of water or as directed by a naturopath

- Black walnut
- Una de Cato
- Echinacea

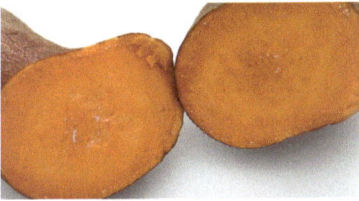

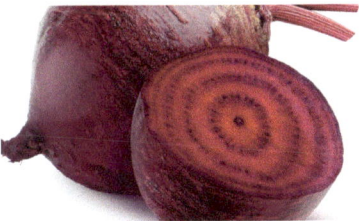

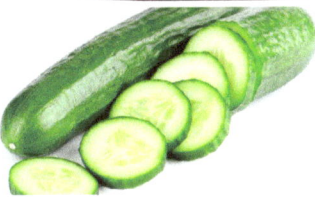

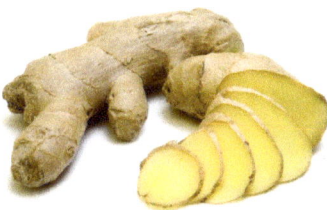

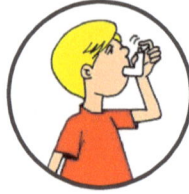

ASTHMA

Asthma is a chronic inflammatory disease of the airways. Asthma is thought to be caused by a combination of genetic and environmental factors and is characterized by wheezing, coughing, chest tightness, and shortness of breath.

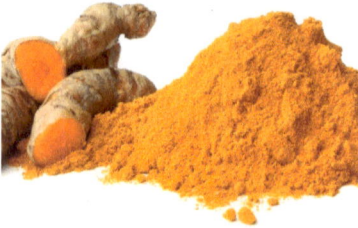

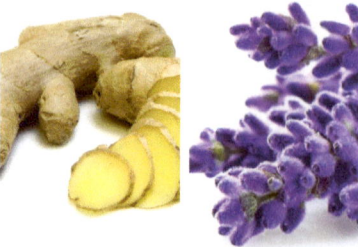

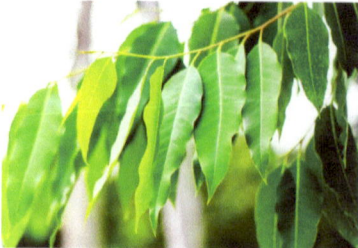

HOMEOPATHIC
- Lobelia Inflata 30c
- Aconite 30c
- Arsenicum album 30c

ESSENTIAL OILS
3 to 4 drops with 25 ml of sweet almond oil and massage into the back.
- Juniper
- Lavender (anti-inflammatory)
- Eucalyptus
- Ginger

VITAMINS
- Vitamin D one a day
- B12 one a day
- Omega-3 one a day

FOODS
- Apples
- Onions
- Dried figs
- Turmeric
- Raw honey
- Carrots
- Ginger

AVOID
- Dairy products (e.g. milk, cheese, butter)
- Fried, fatty foods
- Refined sugars (e.g. white sugar)

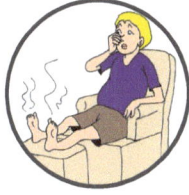

ATHLETE'S FOOT

Athlete's foot is a common fungal infection of the foot. Symptoms include itching, burning, inflammation, and dry cracks in between the toes. Causes are a weakened immune system, or you could pick it up being in public showers and gyms. It is caused by fungi typically transmitted in moist, communal areas where people go barefoot, such as around swimming pools or in locker rooms. These fungi require a warm, moist environment like the inside of a shoe to incubate.

ESSENTIAL OILS

2 drops with 15 ml sweet almond oil and rub on both feet.

- Tea tree
- Calendula
- Geranium

VITAMINS

- Acidophilus take one on an empty stomach
- Zinc take one with food

LIFESTYLE

- Fresh-garlic paste (placed onto foot)
- Baking-soda paste (placed onto foot)
- Black tea (placed onto foot)
- Organic apple cider vinegar soak feet in a foot bath and add 1 big tablespoon

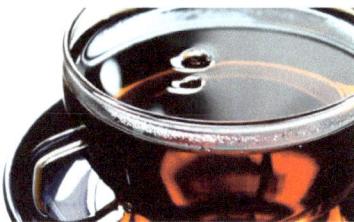

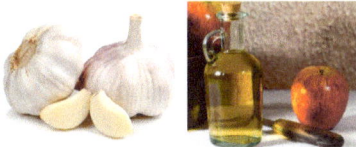

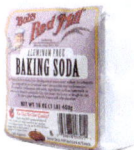

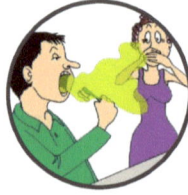

BAD BREATH

Halitosis or chronic bad breath is usually a sign of bacteria in the mouth or a build up of heavy metals. It can be caused by system-ic disease, gastrointestinal disease, and/or respiratory disease. Bad breath can be an indication of a sluggish digestive system.

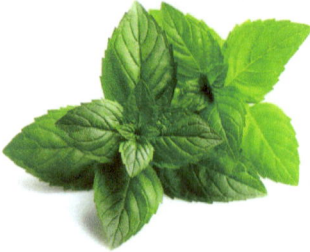

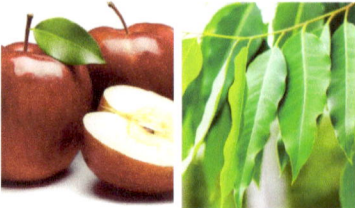

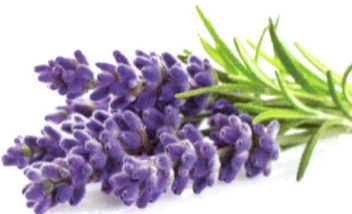

ESSENTIAL OILS
Fill small bottle with 120 ml warm filter water and add 3 drops of oil. Swish mixture in mouth and spit it out afterwards.

- Peppermint oil
- Eucalyptus oil
- Wintergreen
- Lavender

FOODS
- Carrots
- Celery
- Apples
- Alfalfa sprouts
- Water

ORGANIC TEAS
Drink 3 to 4 times a day

- Stinging nettle
- Fennel
- Sage
- Echinacea

LIFESTYLE
- Guava leaf (helps freshen your breath)
- Fresh parsley (chew after each meal)
- Fresh mint (chew after each meal)
- Tongue scraper
- Organic Coconut Oil

AVOID
- Garlic
- Onion
- Refined sugars (e.g. white sugar)
- Alcohol
- Smoking

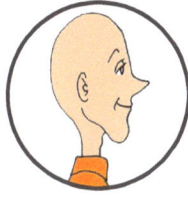

BALDNESS (ALOPECIA)

Baldness (alopecia) is the loss of hair from the head or body. It can have many causes, including a fungal infection, radiotherapy or chemotherapy, and as a result of nutritional deficiencies, such as an iron deficiency. Baldness can also be caused by an autoimmune phenomena, and in males, baldness is both genetic and associated with the male sex hormones called androgens. In some cases, it can also be caused by psychological issues.

HOMEOPATHIC

Once a day

- Thuja 30c
- Folliculinum 6c

ESSENTIAL OILS

Add 3-5 drops of oil in shampoo or with a carrier oil.

- Coconut
- Castor
- Rosemary
- Jojoba (used with carrier oil)
- Basil
- Lemon

VITAMINS

One a day with food

- Kelp
- Biotin
- Vitamin D
- Calcium
- Evening primrose

FOODS

- Walnuts
- Spinach
- Almonds
- Organic salmon
- Sardines
- Lettuce
- Egg yolk
- Flaxseeds

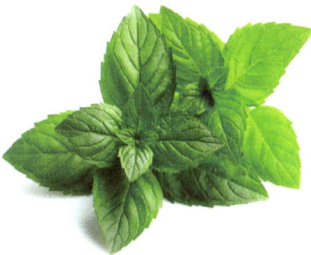

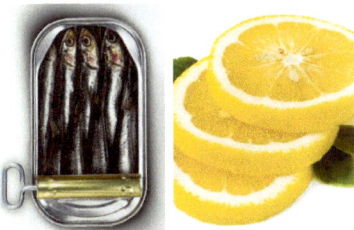

BALDNESS (ALOPECIA)
continued

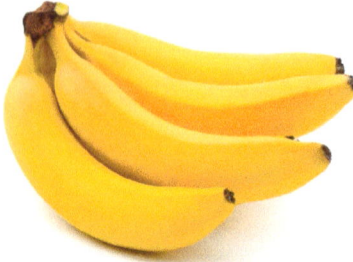

LIFESTYLE

- Aloe vera (applied to open up clogged hair follicles)
- Organic apple-cider vinegar and water (applied to scalp)
- Banana pulp mashed up (applied to scalp)

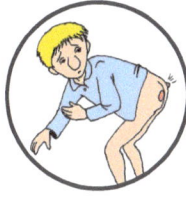

BED SORES

Bedsores are skin lesions caused by medication, age, incapacity, and humidity. Sores are created when skin suffocates beneath the weight of the body. These sores usually occur on bedridden patients.

Any part of the body can be affected. Bedsores can develop and progress rapidly.

HOMEOPATHIC
One twice a day
- Calendula 30c
- Hypericum 30c
- Nat Sulphuricum 30c
- Hamamelis 30c

ESSENTIAL OILS
2 drops in bath
- Tea tree
- Calendula
- Lavender
- Evening primrose

VITAMINS
One a day with food
- Vitamin C
- Zinc
- Aloe vera
- Goldenseal
- Calendula
- Iron
- Arginine

FOODS
- Carrot juice
- Red grape juice

LIFESTYLE
- Honey and sugar (applied on sores)
- Rescue remedy cream (applied on sores)

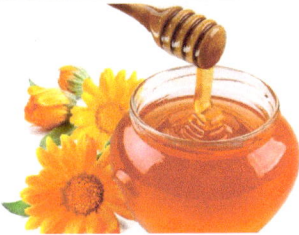

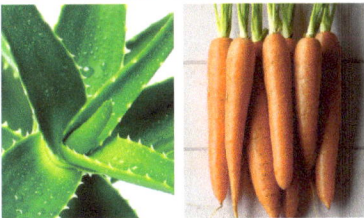

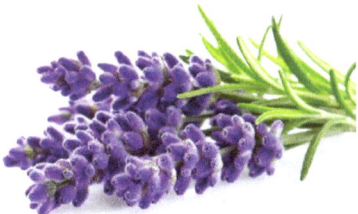

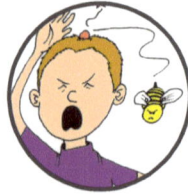

BEE STING

A bee sting is a sting from a honey, bumble, or sweat bee and is quite painful. Bee stings differ from insect bites, and the venom or toxin of stinging insects is quite different. Therefore, the body's reaction to a bee sting may differ significantly from one species to another. In people who are allergic to a sting, a bee sting can trigger an anaphylactic reaction that is potentially dangerous.

HOMEOPATHIC
- Apis mellifica 200c
- Aconite 30c

ESSENTIAL OILS
2 to 3 drops in carrier oil applied on the bee sting
- Lavender
- Parsley

LIFESTYLE
- Apple-cider vinegar
- Baking soda mix in small amount of filter water until paste then apply on bee sting

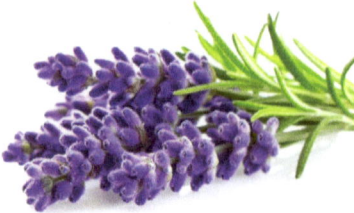

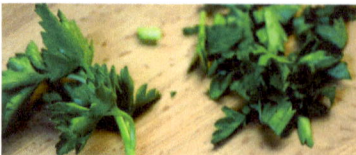

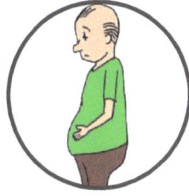

BLOATED STOMACH

Bloated stomachs can often be caused by a very sensitive gut, and certain foods may trigger bloating. There are many causes of bloating, including diet, irritable bowel syndrome, lactose intolerance, reflux, and constipation. Some conditions, such as Crohn's disease or a bowel obstruction, can also contribute to the amount of stomach bloating experienced. Gas and bloating are signs that food is not being digested correctly by the body.

HOMEOPATHIC
Twice a day
- Lycopodium 30c
- Nat-sulp 30c
- Carb Veg 30c
- Colocynthis 6c

VITAMIN
One twice a day
- Enzymes

ESSENTIAL OILS
Massage the stomach in circular motion
- Kava
- Peppermint
- Basil
- Slippery elm
- Cancer bush

FOODS
- Probiotics take one in the morning on an empty stomach
- Fresh lemon in warm water
- Fresh mint
- Ginger
- Bitter cucumber
- Fennel
- Organic Romaine Lettuce
- Organic Bone Broth
- Organic Vegetable Broth

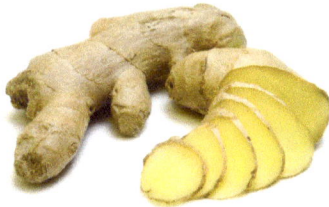

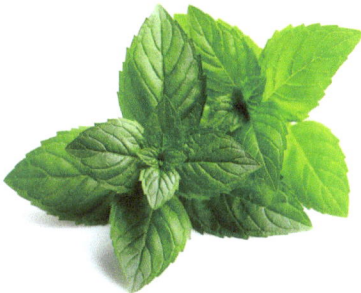

BLOATED STOMACH
continued

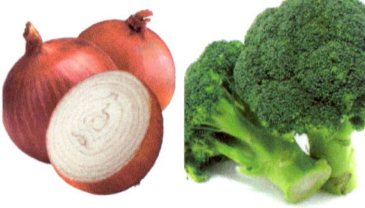

AVOID
- High-salt diet
- Broccoli
- Cauliflower
- Lentils
- Celery
- Onions
- Raisins
- Apricots
- Dairy
- Fats
- Sugar
- Apples

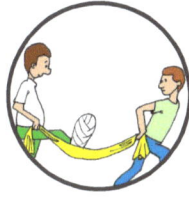

BROKEN FOOT

The human foot contains twenty-six bones. Along with those bones, the foot contains a large network of ligaments, tendons, nerves, and blood vessels. A broken foot can occur as the result of a direct blow, overuse, a severe twist, or a heavy dropped object. The treatment for a broken foot largely depends on the severity of the fracture, but it can include immobilization or surgery.

HOMEOPATHIC
One twice a day
- Carb-Vegetabillis 6c
- Kali-Phos 6c
- Symphytum Officinale 30c
- Arnica 6c
- Ruta graveolens 6c
- Rhus-Toxicodendron 30c

ESSENTIAL OILS
Mix 15 ml of grape seed oil with 1 drop of black pepper and 2 drops of ginger and lavender gently massage in the affected area, and cover it afterward with a warm towel.
- Black pepper
- Ginger
- Lavender
- Turmeric
- Sandalwood
- Myrrh
- Frankincense
- Balsam

VITAMINS
- Calcium take one a day
- Vitamin D take one a day
- Cod liver take one a day
- Bromelain take one a day

FOODS
- Papaya
- Ginger
- Pineapple

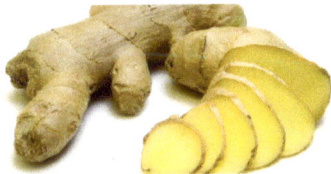

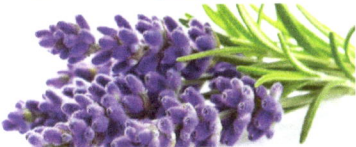

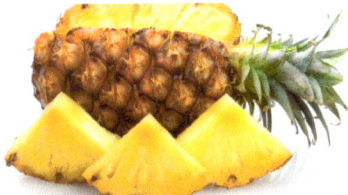

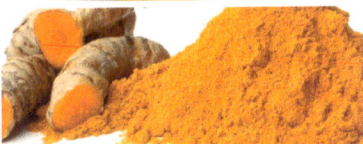

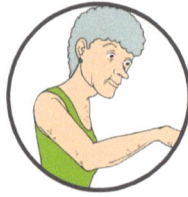

BROWN SPOTS

Brown spots are blemishes that appear on the skin. These spots can appear on the face, hands, scalp, and arms. Causes of brown spots are exposure to ultraviolet light, hormone imbalances, acne, aging, and vitamin B deficiencies.

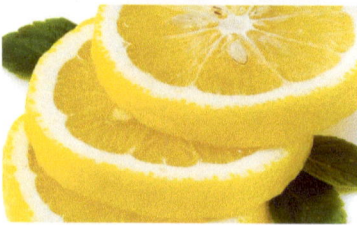

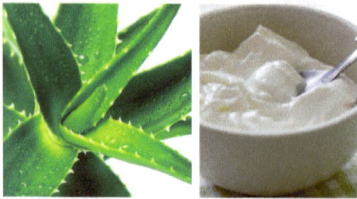

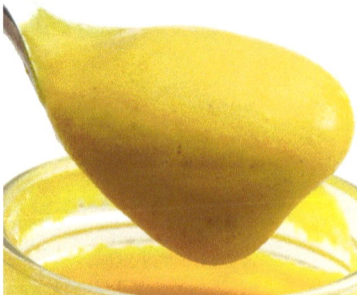

VITAMINS

- Vitamin C one a day
- Vitamin A consult doctor before using
- Vitamin E one a day

ESSENTIAL OILS

Mix a drop of patchouli, lavender with coconut oil. Always test on the skin and dilute during pregnancy to avoid sensitization.

- Patchouli
- Geranium

LIFESTYLE

Food applied onto the brown spots, including:

- Natural yogurt
- Aloe vera juice
- Onion slices
- Lemon
- Yellow mustard
- Horseradish juice

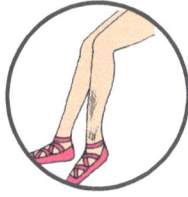

BRUISES

A bruise (contusion) is a type of hematoma of tissue where capillaries and sometimes venules are damaged by trauma, allowing blood to seep, hemorrhage, or extravasate into the surrounding interstitial tissues.

HOMEOPATHY
- Arnica 30c

VITAMINS
- Bromelain one a day
- Vitamin C one a day
- Vitamin E one a day
- Zinc one a day after food

FOODS
- Pineapples

LIFESTYLE
- Arnica cream
- Parsley compress
- Onion compress on the areas
- Organic Apple-cider vinegar compress

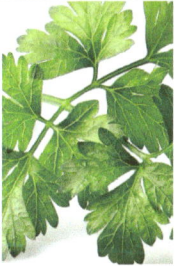

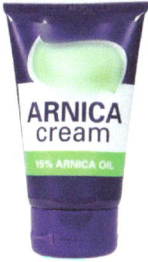

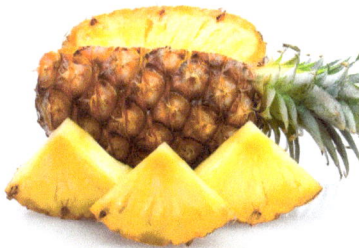

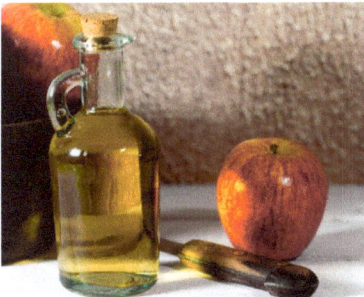

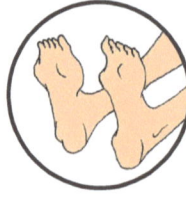

BUNIONS

A bunion is an abnormal formation in the bones of the big-toe joint. These lumps prevent a regular shoe from fitting properly and can cause significant pain.

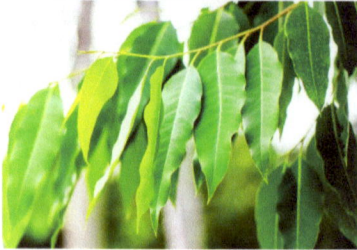

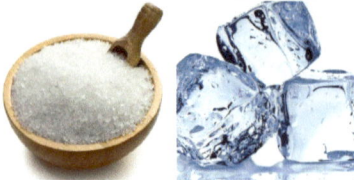

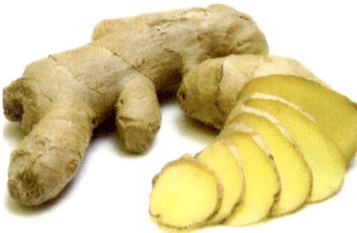

HOMEOPATHIC

- Arnica 30c
- Sulphur 30c

ESSENTIAL OILS

Mix 10ml of sweet almond oil, 3 drops of eucalyptus, ginger and one drop of wintergreen. Massage into the bunions.

- Lemongrass
- Wintergreen
- Eucalyptus
- Ginger

VITAMINS

- Capsicum one a day

GENERAL

- Calendula
- Tiger balm
- Epsom salt
- Ice pack
- Bunion splint

AVOID

- High heels

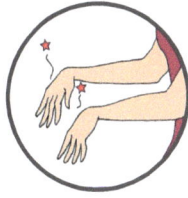

CARPAL TUNNEL

Carpal tunnel is a painful, progressive condition that occurs when the median nerve in the wrist is compressed. Carpal tunnel causes numbness, tingling, and pain in the hands and fingers.

HOMEOPATHIC

- Arnica 30c
- Rhus toxicodendron 30c

VITAMINS

- Bromelaine one a day
- Vitamin B12 one a day
- Vitamin B6 one a day
- Lipoic acid one a day

FOODS

- Pineapples
- Papaya
- Salmon
- Ginger
- Sweet potatoes
- Wild yam

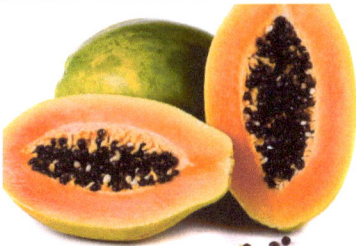

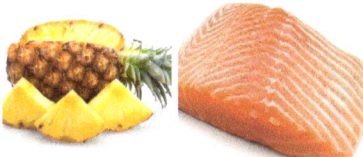

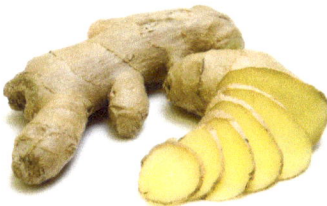

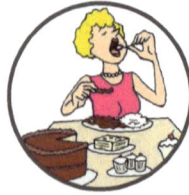

CHOLESTEROL

Cholesterol is an organic, lipid molecule essential to maintaining both cell membrane structural integrity and fluidity. In addition to its importance within cells, cholesterol also serves as a precursor for the biosynthesis of steroid hormones, bile acids, and vitamin D. Although cholesterol is important, high levels increase the risk of heart attack and stroke.

ESSENTIAL OILS

4 drops each of peppermint, lavender and lemon grass oil daily.

- Peppermint
- Lavender
- Lemongrass

VITAMINS

- Vitamin B3 one a day
- Artichoke leaf one a day
- Garlic one a day

FOODS

- Oats
- Barley
- Carrots
- Brussels sprouts
- Flaxseeds
- Yam
- Celery

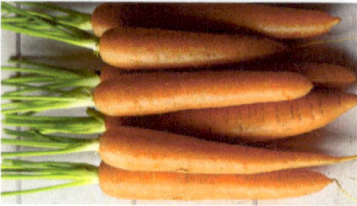

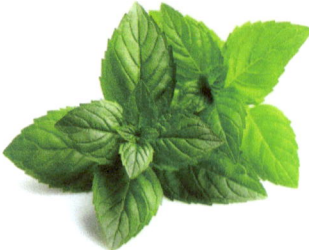

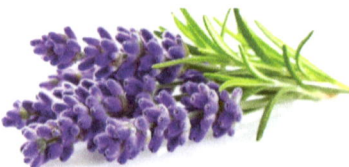

HERBAL TEAS

- Green tea 3 to 4 cups a day with water to ensure adequate hydration

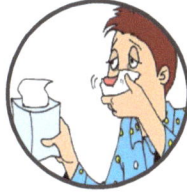

COLDS and FLU

The common cold is a viral infection of the upper respiratory tract (nose and throat). A common cold is usually harmless, although it may not feel that way. If it is not a runny nose, sore throat, and cough, it is the watery eyes, sneezing, and congestion—or maybe all the above. In fact, more than 100 viruses can cause a common cold, so signs and symptoms tend to vary greatly.

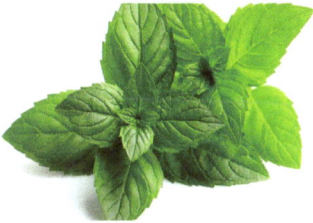

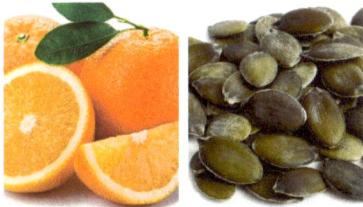

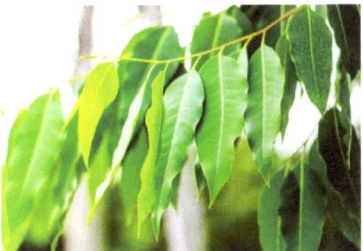

HOMEOPATHIC
Start taking Aconite, then Oscilloccinum once a day and Allium Cepa 3 times a day

- Aconite 6c
- Gelsemium 30c
- Oscillococcinum 200c
- Allium Cepa 6c

VITAMINS
- Vitamin C twice a day
- Colloidal Silver 1 dropper in the morning

ESSENTIAL OILS
3 drops of eucalyptus oil, 1 drop of pine and 1 drop of cinnamon in diffuser

- Eucalyptus
- Pine
- Cinnamon

FOODS
- Oranges
- Garlic
- Pumpkin
- Mustard seeds
- Kiwi

HERBS
- Ginger drink once a day
- Peppermint drink twice a day
- Chamomile drink 3 times a day
- Echinacea 10 drops in 8oz of water

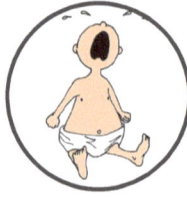

COLIC

Colic is a form of pain that starts and stops abruptly. It occurs due to muscular contractions of a hollow tube (colon, ureter, gall bladder, etc.) in an attempt to relieve the obstruction by forcing content out. It may be accompanied by vomiting and sweating. Colic often occurs in babies and can cause crying/uncontrolled screaming, which stems in part from gastrointestinal discomfort.

HOMEOPATHIC
- Colocynthis 30c
- Chamomilla 30c
- Nux vomica 30c
- Lycopodium 30c

VITAMINS
- Probiotics on an empty stomach
- Digestive enzymes one a day
- Peppermint capsules take twice a day

ESSENTIAL OILS
15ml of Sweet Almond oil, 4 drops of peppermint oil and 2 drops of chamomile oil. Massage into the stomach.
- Chamomile oil
- Peppermint oil

HERBAL TEAS:
Drink up to 3/4 cups a day
- Chamomile
- Aniseed
- Fresh peppermint

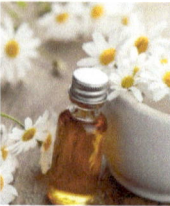

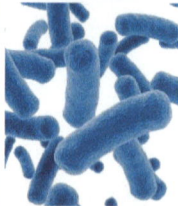

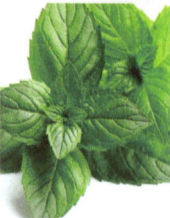

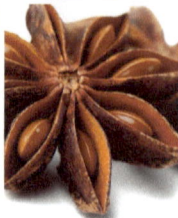

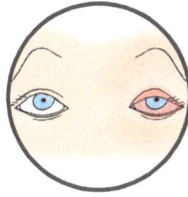

CONJUNCTIVITIS

Conjunctivitis is the inflammation of the membrane covering the inside of your eyelid. It is commonly caused by an infection (usually viral, but sometimes bacterial), or it can be the result of an allergic reaction.

HOMEOPATHIC
- Euphrasia 6c take twice a day
- Argentum Nitricum 6c take once a day
- Apis Mellifica 6c take once a day
- Pulsatilla Nigricans 6c take twice day

VITAMINS
- Vitamin C one a day
- Elderberry tincture take 10 drops with 8 oz of filter water
- Zinc take one a day with food

HERBAL TEAS
Drink up to 4 cups a day
- Raspberry
- Comfrey root
- Chamomile

LIFESTYLE
- Chamomile tea bags soaked in warm water applied to the infected area

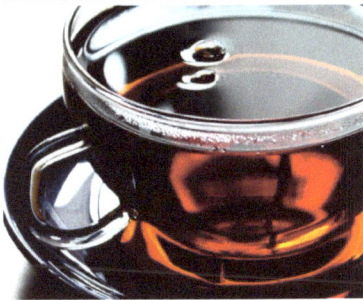

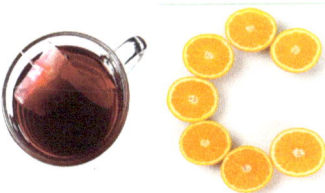

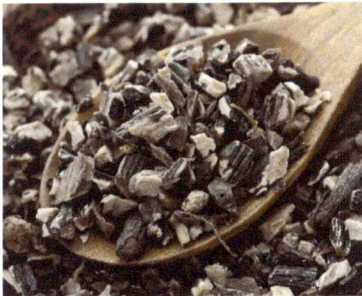

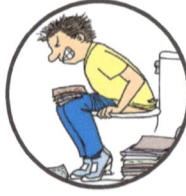

CONSTIPATION

Constipation is infrequent bowel movements that are hard to pass. Usually, constipation is not life threatening but can make you feel bloated and uncomfortable. In severe cases, a bowel obstruction can become life-threatening.

HOMEOPATHIC
Take up to twice a day
- Nux Vomica 30c
- Bryonia 30c
- Arg-Nitricum 30c

FOODS
- Rhubarb
- Aloe
- Orange juice with a tablespoon of olive oil
- Warm glass of lemon in the morning
- Figs (dry or fresh)
- Flaxseeds
- Spinach
- Oranges
- Plenty of water
- Add more fiber to your diet

LIFESTYLE
- Yoga
- Exercise (cardio-based)

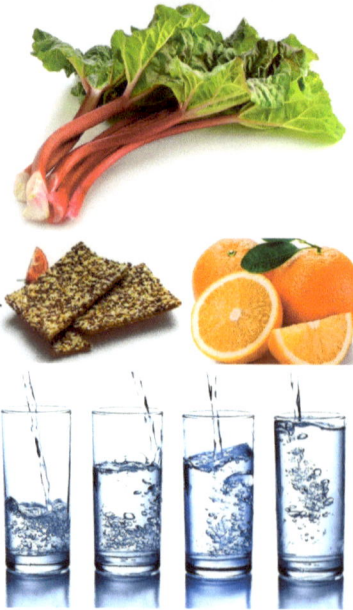

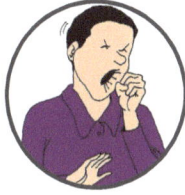

COUGH

Coughing is a natural reflex to help clear out foreign particles, irritants, and secretions from our lungs and airways. The forced and sometimes violent exhalation can be voluntary as well as reflexive. Coughing is useful for moving and clearing out anything disturbing our breathing from the respiratory system. Coughs can be spasmodic as your body tries to eliminate the mucus.

HOMEOPATHIC
- Aconite 30c 1 to 3 a day depending on the cough
- Bryonia 6c 3 x a day
- Drosera 30c twice a day
- Arnica 6c once a day
- Phosphorus 30c once a day

ESSENTIAL OILS
3 to 4 drops of ginger, eucalyptus and 2 drops of lemon mixed into 25ml carrier oil in hot bath
- Lemon
- Eucalyptus
- Pine

VITAMINS
- Vitamin C one a day
- Zinc one a day after meals

HERBS
- Slippery elm
- Elderberry

FOODS
- Chicken soup
- Dark chocolate
- Apple-cider vinegar
- Spicy soups
- Oranges
- Kiwis
- Bell peppers
- Broccoli

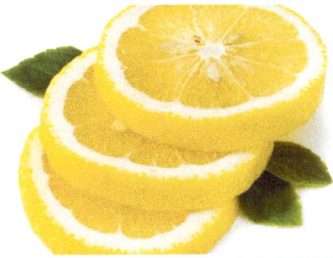

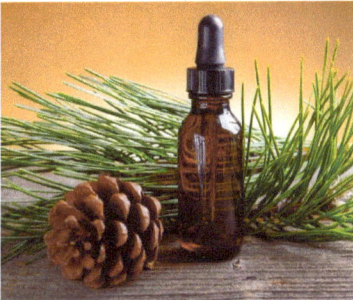

COUGH
continued

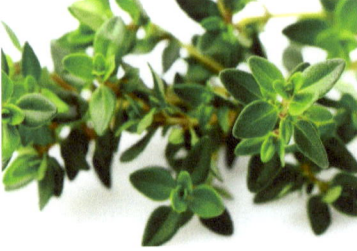

HERBAL TEAS
- Garlic
- Mullein
- Thyme
- Rose water

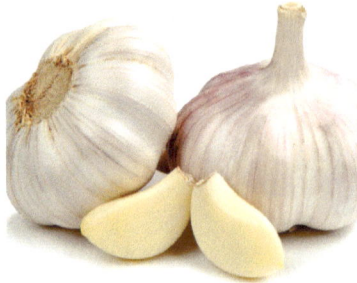

AVOID
- Grapes
- Dairy (e.g. milk, butter, cheese)

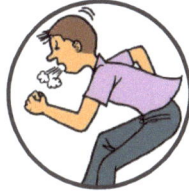

CROUP

Croup is a virus that presents itself as a barking cough. Croup is an infection of the upper airway; children are very prone to getting croup.

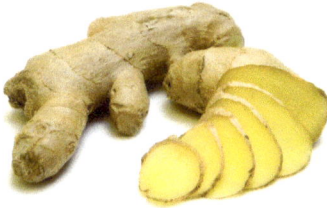

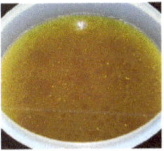

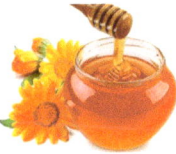

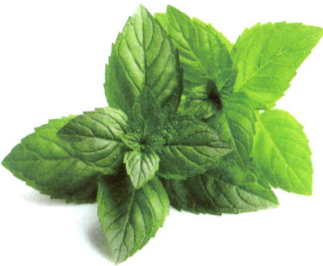

HOMEOPATHIC

- Drosera 6c
- Spongia Tosta 30c
- Antimonium Crudum 30c
- Aconite 6c

ESSENTIAL OILS

3 drops eucalyptus oil and 2 drops of peppermint oil mixed with 20ml of carrier oil and apply to chest and upper back.

- Eucalyptus
- Peppermint

FOODS

- Chicken broth
- Warm foods, especially hearty soups
- Ginger
- Honey
- Apple-cider vinegar

HERBAL TEAS

- Chamomile
- Peppermint
- Ginger

LIFESTYLE

- Hot showers or a bath can also help.

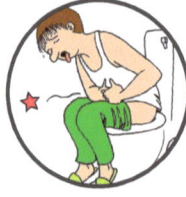

DIARRHEA

Diarrhea is the body's cleansing response, removing unwanted substances through digestive tract looseness.

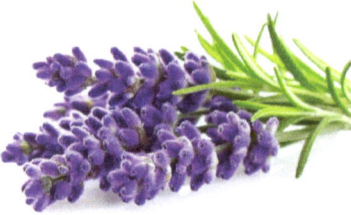

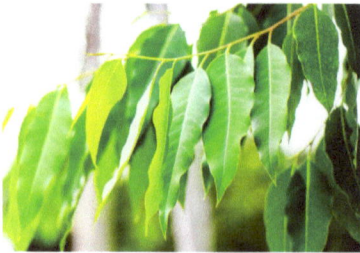

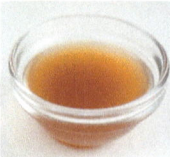

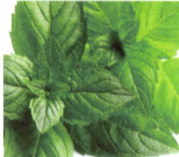

HOMEOPATHIC
- Podophyllum Peltatum 6c as directed
- Sulphur 6c once a day
- Arsenicum Album 6c once a day

ESSENTIAL OILS
4 drops of lavender and geranium mixed with 20ml of carrier oil. Massage the abdomen in clockwise direction.
- Peppermint
- Lavender
- Chamomile
- Eucalyptus
- Geranium

FOODS
- Rice
- Bananas
- Guava
- Apples
- Apple-cider vinegar
- Dry crackers
- Plenty of fluids (e.g. water)

AVOID
- Dairy (e.g. milk, cheese, butter)
- Caffeine
- Alcohol
- Fatty foods

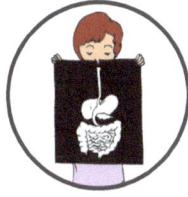

DIGESTION

Digestion problems can be caused by anxiety, stress and tension. Also some foods, your body can't digest, can cause problems with digestion.

HOMEOPATHIC
One every 15-30 minutes
- Carbo Vegetabilis 30c
- Colocynthis 30c
- Nux Vomica 30c
- Lycopodium 30c

ESSENTIAL OILS
- Peppermint
- Chamomile
- Lemon balm
- Fennel
- Ginger Root
- Herbal teas (e.g. peppermint, licorice)

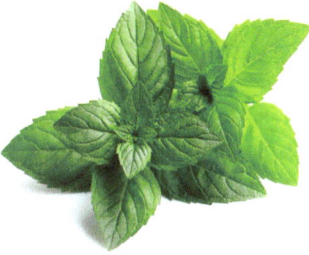

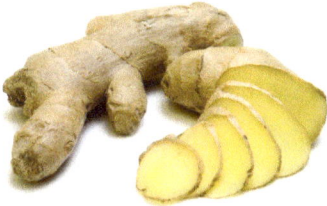

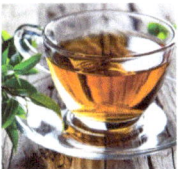

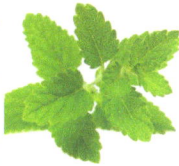

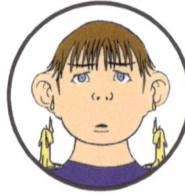

EARWAX BUILDUP

Earwax is part of the body's immune system; it protects the inner ear by preventing bacteria from entering it. Earwax blockage occurs when earwax accumulates in the ear because it cannot be drained away. Earwax blockage, can be associated with a number of symptoms, including ringing in the ears, ear pain, dizziness, and decreased hearing.

Earwax is a self-cleaning agent with protective lubricating and antibacterial properties.

Using a cotton swab to clean earwax can cause the build-up of earwax and can block the ear canal.

HOMEOPATHIC
- Aconite 30c (first onset)
- Pulsatilla nigricans 6c
- Chamomilla vulg 6c
- Kali-muriaticum 6x (cell salt)
- Hepar-sulphuris 6c
- Silica marina 6c

ESSENTIAL OILS
Apply to external ear
- Almond
- Mullein
- Eucalyptus
- Coconut
- Lavender
- Olive

LIFESTYLE
- Organic apple-cider vinegar
- Salt water helps remove earwax
- Hydrogen peroxide

AVOID
- Dairy (e.g. milk, cheese, butter)
- Wheat
- Eggs
- Corn

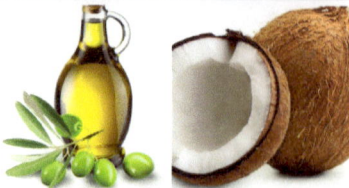

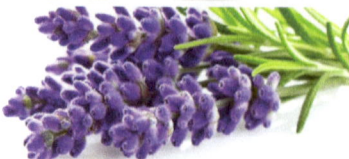

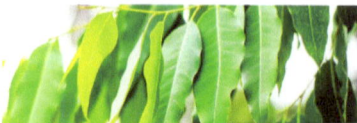

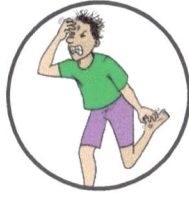

ECZEMA

Eczema is an irritating skin disease in which the skin develops areas of itchy, scaly rashes. It is very common in younger children but can also affect older people. It is also known as topic dermatitis, which is a chronic allergic condition and is caused by a combination of hereditary and environmental factors. Eczema commonly affects the face, scalp, elbows, hands, and knees. Blisters on the skin can also form as a result of scratching. Certain detergents, dust mites, and animal dander can trigger eczema.

HOMEOPATHIC

- Apis 6c
- Histaminum 30c
- Sepia 6c
- Ledum 6c
- Urtica urens 6c
- Rhus Tox 30c
- Arsenicum 30c
- Graphites 30c
- Mezereum 30c
- Nat Mur 30c

ESSENTIAL OILS

2 drops combined with a tablespoon of coconut oil. Rub into feet.

- Coconut
- Borage
- Magnesium
- Vitamin E
- Sage
- Sweet marjoram
- Frankincense
- Myrrh
- Spike lavender
- German chamomile

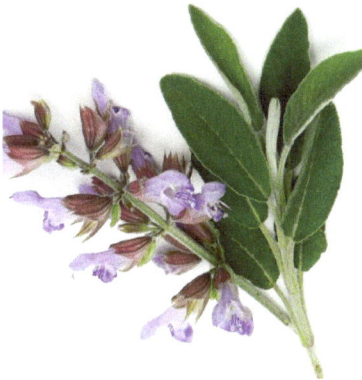

ECZEMA
continued

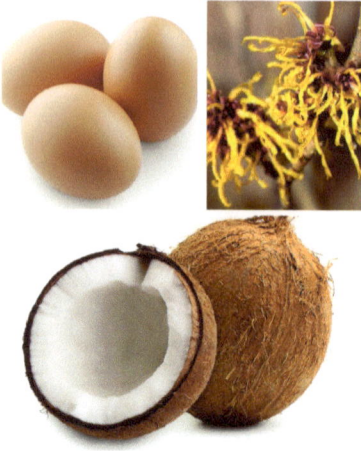

LIFESTYLE

- Egg white applied on the affected skin
- Sulphur cream
- Aloe vera gel
- Calendula lotion
- Seven cream
- Oatmeal bath – place oatmeal in a sock and leave in the bath
- Magnesium bath
- Aluminium-free baking-soda bath
- Organic apple-cider vinegar
- Chamomile
- Witch hazel
- Licorice
- Himalayan salt (with added warm-water compress)

AVOID

- Alcohol
- Items that contain caffeine

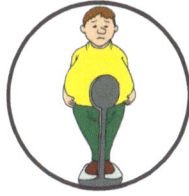

EDEMA

Edema is swelling of the body, where fluid becomes stuck in the tissues, usually in the extremities (such as feet, hands, and face). Certain medications can also cause it.

HOMEOPATHIC
One two times daily

- Apis 30c
- Calcarea Carbonica 6c

VITAMINS
Take with food daily

- Quercetin
- Probiotics one on a empty stomach
- Fish oils (EPA)
- Evening primrose
- Bromelain
- Flavonoids
- Alpha lipoid acid

FOODS

- Whole grains
- Dark, leafy greens
- Spinach kale
- Sea vegetables
- Asparagus
- Parsley
- Beets
- Pineapple

HERBS
10 drops in 8oz water

- Bilberry
- Dandelion
- Grape-seed extract
- Milk thistle
- Galium Aparine
- Horsetail plant
- Cornsilk
- Horse Chestnut

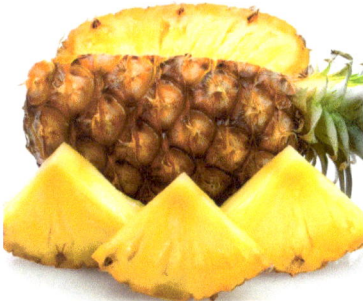

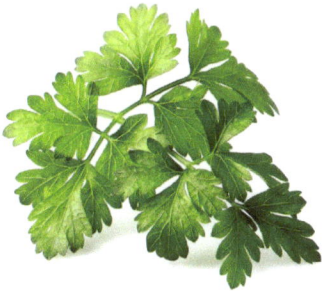

EDEMA
continued

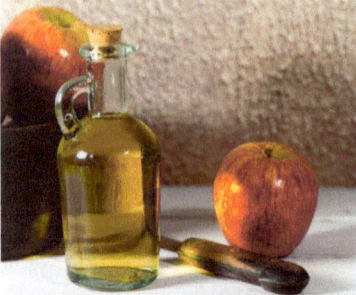

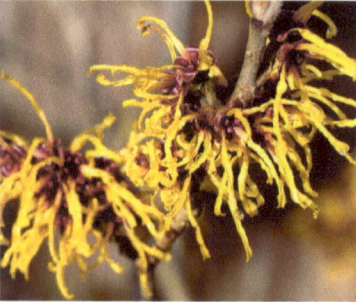

HERBAL TEAS

- Yarrow
- Dandelion

LIFESTYLE

- Organic blackstrap molasses 1 tablespoon in 5oz warm hemp milk
- Organic apple-cider vinegar
- Chickweed cream
- Marigold cream
- Witch hazel
- St. John's Wort cream

AVOID

- Dairy
- Soy
- Corn
- Wheat
- Salt
- Red meats
- Alcohol
- Processed food
- Sugars
- Scratching (apply ice)
- Dust or sand
- Cigarette smoke
- Air pollution
- Heat

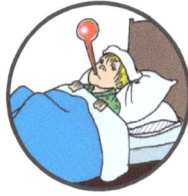

FEVER

Fever (also known as pyrexia) is defined as a body temperature above the normal range due to an increase in the temperature regulatory set-point. Many alternative therapies disagree with some allopathic doctors' belief that a fever should be suppressed. Instead, these therapies hold that a fever is the body's way of fending off an infection, a process that should be allowed to run its course.

HOMEOPATHIC

Try aconite initially every hour and then Belladonna every one to two hours

- Aconite 6c First sign of onset.
- Belladonna 30c
- Nux Vomica 6c
- Pulsatilla Nigricans 30c
- Ferrum Phosphoricum 6c

ESSENTIAL OILS

5 drops with 25ml sweet almond oil. Massage into the neck, chest and soles of feet.

- Chamomile
- Black pepper
- Peppermint
- Hyssop
- Lemon
- Tea tree

FOODS

- Chicken soup

LIFESTYLE

- Bathing with 1 tablespoon apple-cider vinegar
- Probiotics

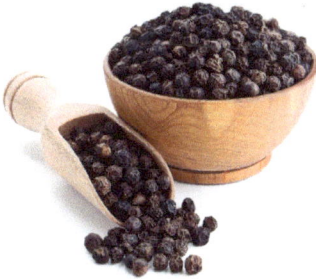

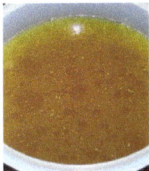

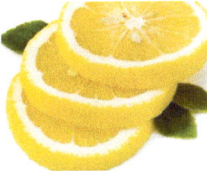

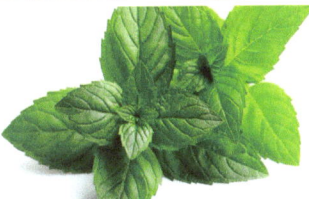

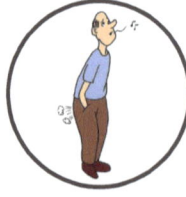

FLATULENCE

Most intestinal gas comes from swallowed air (e.g., when sipping a drink) or is due to bacterial action in the intestine. Flatulence is composed of many different gases, including carbon dioxide, oxygen, nitrogen, and methane.

HOMEOPATHIC
One dose four times a day.
- Carbo Veg 200c
- Lycopodium 30c
- China Officinalis 30c

FOODS
- Cinnamon
- Peppermint
- Fennel
- Cardamom
- Lemon balm
- Papaya
- Pineapple
- Mustard seeds

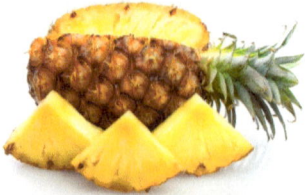

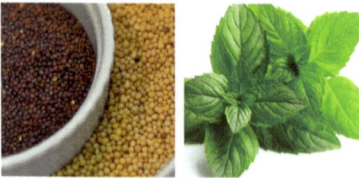

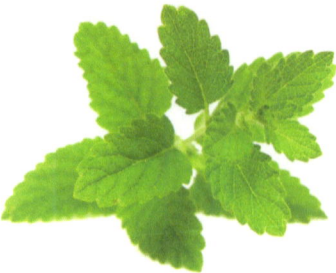

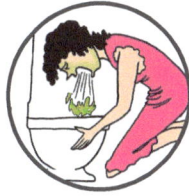

FOOD POISONING

Food poisoning is caused by eating contaminated food. Food can become contaminated by infection or toxin, and when ingested can lead to nausea and diarrhoea. Some cases of food poisoning may require hospitalization.

HOMEOPATHIC
One dose every 2-4 hours.

- Arsenicum Album 30c
- Podophyllum 30c

FOODS
- Apple-cider vinegar
- Ginger
- Cumin
- Basil
- Bananas
- Apples
- Lemon
- Activated charcoal
- Water

HERBAL TEAS
drink 4 times a day

- Peppermint

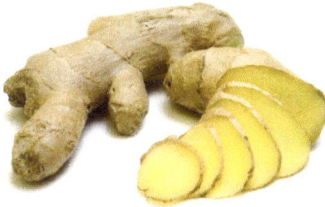

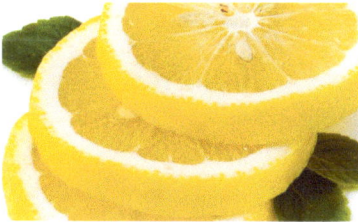

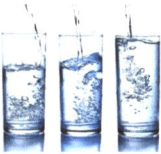

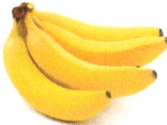

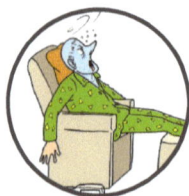

HANGOVER

A hangover is the experience of the effects following the consumption of alcohol. Typical symptoms of a hangover may include headache, drowsiness, concentration problems, dry mouth, dizziness, fatigue, gastrointestinal distress, sweating, nausea, hyper-excitability, and anxiety.

HOMEOPATHIC
Take one every ten to thirty minutes
- Nux Vomica 6c
- Chelidonium 3x

ESSENTIAL OILS
Add 3 drops to 80ml filtered water and diffuse
- Peppermint
- Lemongrass
- Lavender

VITAMINS
Take one a day with food
- Vitamin C
- Probiotic take one om empty stomach
- Zinc

FOODS
- Lemon in water
- Fresh ginger
- Fresh coconut water
- Hearty breakfast

AVOID
- Alcohol

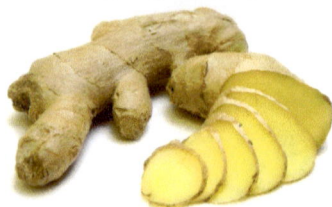

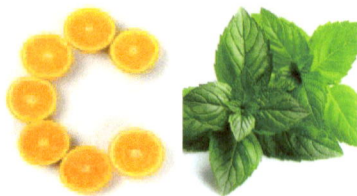

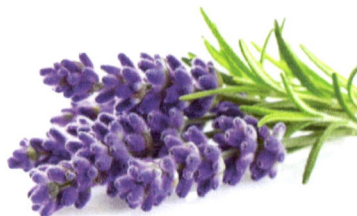

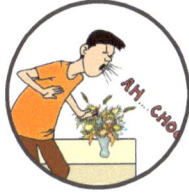

HAY FEVER

Hay fever (allergic rhinitis) is inflammation of the nasal airways caused by an allergic reaction. It occurs when an allergen, such as pollen, is inhaled by someone who is sensitized to that allergen. Hay fever symptoms resemble a cold or flu.

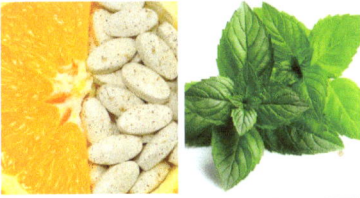

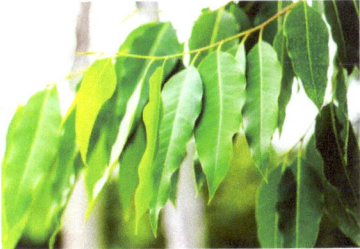

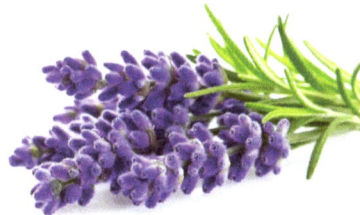

HOMEOPATHIC
One dose up to 4 times a day

- Nux Vomica 6c
- Nat Muriaticum 6c
- Arsenicum Album 6c
- Mixed Pollen 30c
- Histamine 30c

ESSENTIAL OILS
10 drops into bath water.

- Eucalyptus
- Lemon
- Peppermint
- Rosemary
- Lavender

VITAMINS
As directed

- Vitamin C
- Quercetin
- Omega-3 fatty acid

FOODS

- Ginger
- Garlic
- Honey

HERBS
10 drops in water

- Stinging nettle
- Quercetin
- Ginkgo

HAY FEVER
continued

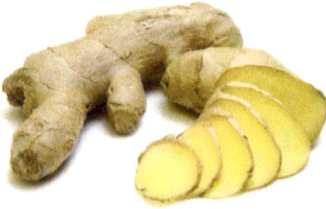

HERBAL TEAS
Drink upto 4 cups a day.
- Chamomile
- Ginger
- Green
- Peppermint

LIFESTYLE
- Butterbur
- Grapefruit and lemon

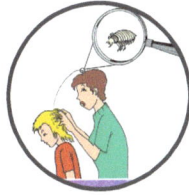

HEAD LICE

Head lice are tiny insects that live on the human body and feed on blood from the scalp.

HOMEOPATHIC
Twice a day
- Staph 30c
- Aconite 30c

ESSENTIAL OILS
5-20 drops of tea tree oil lavender and rosemary in carrier oil. Apply on to hair near scalp
- Lavender
- Rosemary
- Garlic
- Tea tree

LIFESTYLE
- Wash hair with 1 tablespoon organic apple-cider vinegar and 150z water.

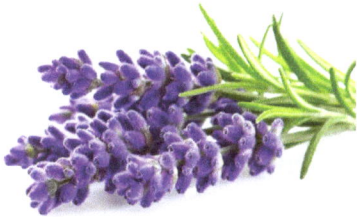

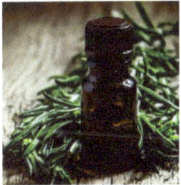

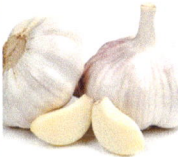

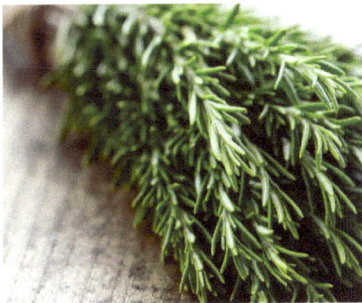

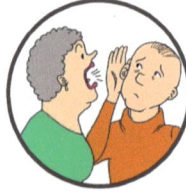

HEARING LOSS

Hearing loss is a partial or total inability to hear. Hearing loss is caused by many factors, including genetics, age, exposure to noise, illness, chemicals, and physical trauma.

HOMEOPATHIC
Three times a day

- Kali Muriaticum 6x
- Kali Sulphuricum 6x
- Natrum Phos 6x
- Causticum 30c
- Belladonna 30c

VITAMINS
One with food

- Vitamin A consult with doctor before taking
- Vitamin C
- Vitamin E

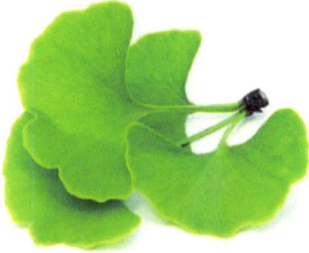

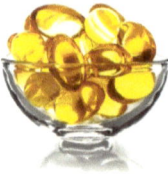

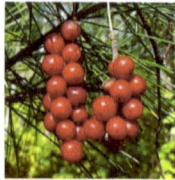

HERBS

- Schizandra herb
- Mullein
- Ginkgo biloba
- Alpha lipoic acid
- N-acetylcysteine (helps protect hair cells in inner ear)

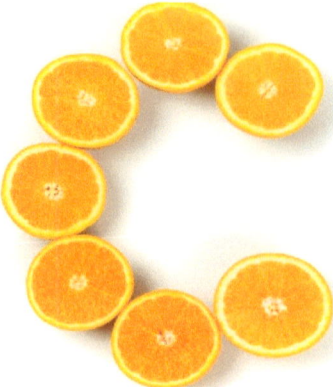

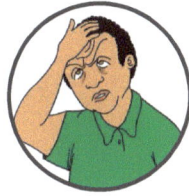

HEADACHES

A headache is caused by dysfunctional pain in your head. A headache is not always a symptom of an underlying disease. Chemical activity in your brain, the nerves or blood vessels of your head outside your skull, or muscles of your head and neck, or some combination of these factors may play a role in primary headaches.

HOMEOPATHIC

One every 15-30 minutes

- Arnica 30c
- Belladonna 30c
- Bryonia Alba 30c
- Cimicifuga 30c
- Gelsemium 30c
- Natrum Muriaticum 30c
- Nux Vomica 30c

ESSENTIAL OILS

1 drop mixed with 5ml of carrier oil. Massage temples and the nape of the neck.

- Peppermint
- Eucalyptus
- Lavender

FOODS

- Yogurt

HERBAL TEAS

Drink upto 3 /4 cups a day

- Ginger
- Roman chamomile

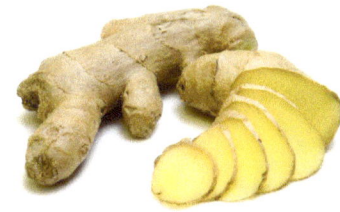

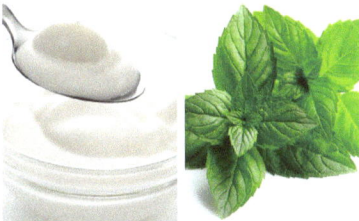

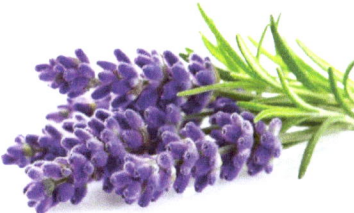

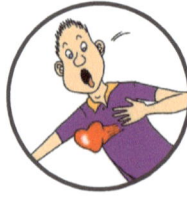

HEART PALPITATIONS

Palpitations are an abnormality of the heartbeat characterized by awareness of heart muscle contractions in the chest: hard beats, fast beats, irregular beats, and/or pauses. Palpitations can be caused by anxiety and do not necessarily indicate an abnormality of the heart. Palpitations can be intermittent or sometimes continuous. Associated symptoms include dizziness, shortness of breath, sweating, headaches, and chest pain.

HOMEOPATHIC
One every 15-30 minutes for 2-3 doses.

- Arsenicum Album 6c
- Aconite 6c

ESSENTIAL OILS
1 drop of each mixed in 20ml carrier oil. Massaged the chest and back

- Chamomile
- Geranium
- Lavender

FOODS
- Grape juice
- Honey

AVOID
- Caffeine
- Chocolate
- Excessive salt

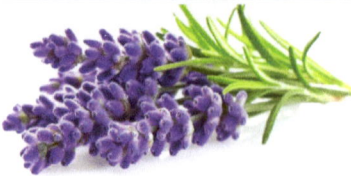

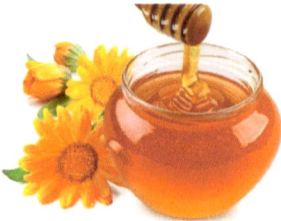

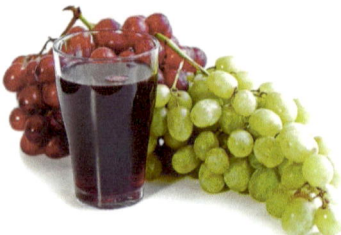

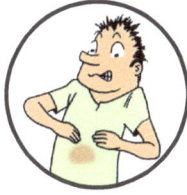

HEARTBURN

Heartburn is a burning feeling in the chest after eating or waking up first thing in the morning, especially after lying down. Heartburn is usually associated with regurgitation of gastric acid.

HOMEOPATHIC
One dose at intervals of 15-30 minutes for 2-3 doses
- Nux Vomica 6 c
- Arsenicum Album 6c

VITAMINS
- Vitamin D once a day with food
- Probiotics one before food

HERBS
- Hydrochloric acid supplement
- Basil leaves
- Caraway
- German chamomile
- Licorice
- Milk thistle
- Peppermint
- Aloe vera juice
- Apple-cider vinegar
- Cinnamon
- Cardamom
- Ginger
- Yellow mustard

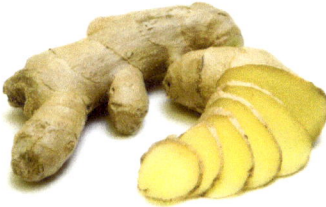

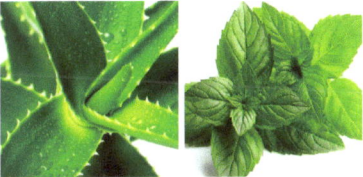

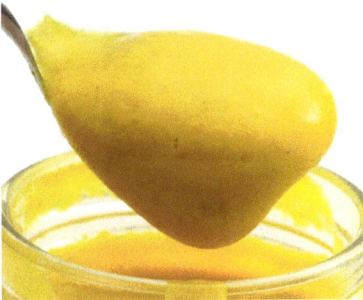

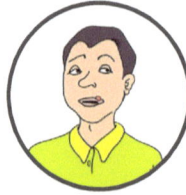

HERPES

Herpes is a common and usually mild recurrent skin condition; most infections are unrecognized and un-diagnosed. Herpes is caused by a virus, the herpes simplex virus (HSV).

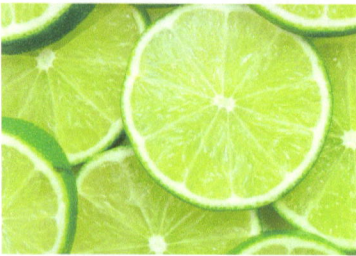

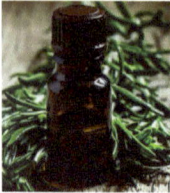

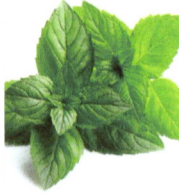

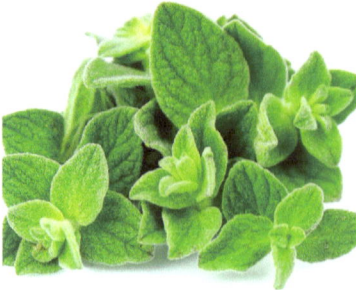

HOMEOPATHIC

3 times a day at the first sign of itch or tingling.

- Rhus Toxicodendron 6c
- Nof Mur 30c

ESSENTIAL OILS

Adding 1 drop of an individual oil or a combination of oils to the affected area 3-4 times a day.

- Oregano
- Tea tree
- Lysine olive leaf extract
- Echinacea

VITAMINS

- Lysine take one a day

FOODS

- I tablespoon of Lime, half tsp ginger juice, and tsp honey mixed in a 8oz glass of warm water
- Aniseed
- Green or herbal tea
- Peppermint
- Baking soda half a spoon mixed with a small amount of water to make a paste and apply on the sore.

LIFESTYLE

- Domeboro Powder—mixed with water can help stop itching, dry the sore, and speed healing

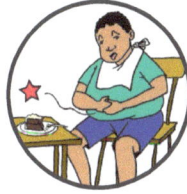

INDIGESTION

Indigestion and gas can be caused by poor eating habits, emotional tension, food allergies, imbalances in stomach acid or digestive enzymes, and many other causes.

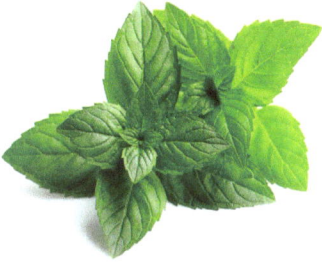

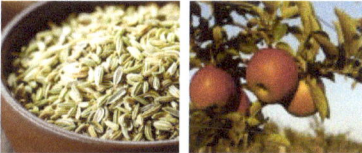

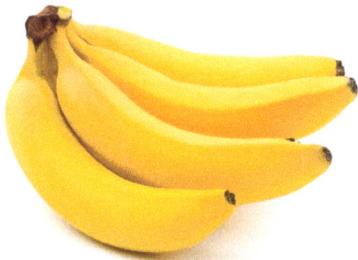

HOMEOPATHIC

One dose at interval of 15-30 minutes for 2-3 doses

- Nux vomica 6c
- Lycopodium 30c

ESSENTIAL OILS

8-10 drops in a bath

- Peppermint
- Fennel

FOODS

- Apples
- Bananas
- Steamed greens
- Fennel seeds
- Cabbage juice
- Peppermint leaves

HERBAL TEAS

Drink up to 3-4 cups a day

- Peppermint

AVOID

- Big meals
- Lying down after eating
- Smoking
- Fatty foods
- Fried foods
- Citrusy fruits
- Alcohol
- Caffeine
- Carbonated drinks

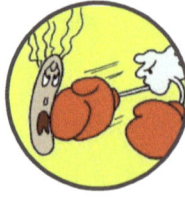

IMMUNE SYSTEM

The immune system is one of the most important systems of the body. A weak immune system causes frequent colds, flu, and chronic illnesses.

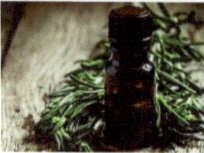

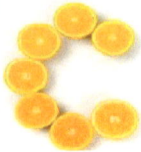

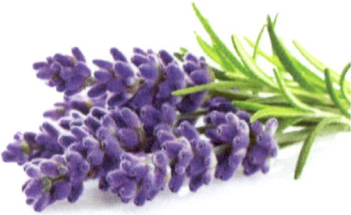

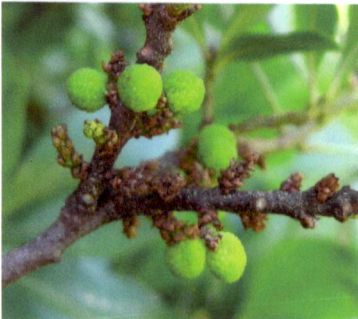

ESSENTIAL OILS
Put 10 drops of lavender 2 drops tea tree and one drop of bergamot in the bath
- Lavender
- Bergamot
- Tea tree

VITAMINS
Take one with food
- Vitamin C
- Zinc
- Echinacea

HERBS
10 drops in 10oz of water
- Astragalus
- Bayberry
- Golden seal

AVOID
- Caffeine

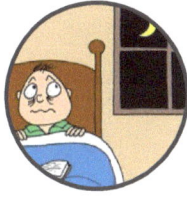

INSOMNIA

Insomnia is the inability to get the amount of sleep you need to wake up feeling rested and refreshed. Because different people need different amounts of sleep, insomnia is defined by the quality of your sleep and how you feel after sleeping, not the number of hours you sleep or how quickly you doze off. Even if you are spending eight hours a night in bed, if you feel drowsy and fatigued during the day, you may be experiencing insomnia.

HOMEOPATHIC
One dose to be taken every evening .Stop with improvements.

- Coffea cruda30c
- Chamomilla 30c

ESSENTIAL OILS
8 drops and soak in the bath before you sleep.

- Lavender
- Chamomilla

VITAMINS
One of the below half a hour before you sleep.

- Melatonin
- l-Tryptophan
- 5-HTP
- Calms forte
- Magnesium

FOODS

- Valeria and Kava calming tea
- Crackers

LIFESTYLE

- Lavender bath in the evening
- Keep bedroom cool
- Avoid leaving electrical devices on
- Acupuncture
- Massage
- Meditation

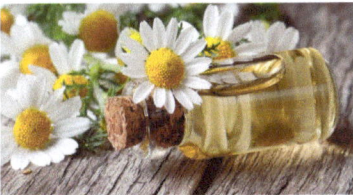

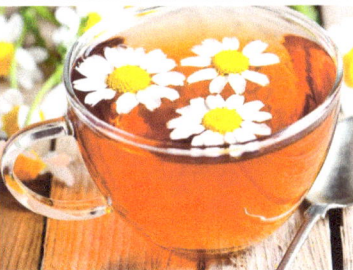

INSOMNIA
continued

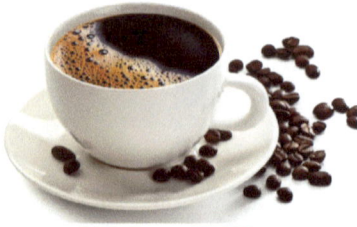

AVOID

- Sweets
- Caffeine
- Naps in the daytime
- Refined foods (e.g. white sugar, bread, rice, cakes, etc)
- Avoid TVs in room

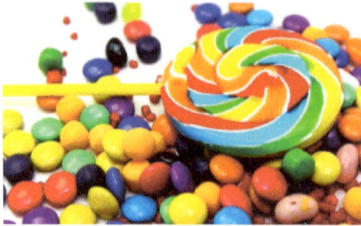

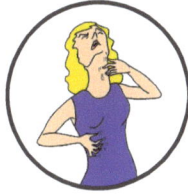

ITCHING

Itching is a sensation that causes the desire to scratch. Itching can be caused by a number of different reasons, including stress and anxiety.

HOMEOPATHIC

One dose on alternate days for a week and then stop with improvement.

- Sulphur 30c
- Arsenicum Album 30c

ESSENTIAL OILS

- Calendula
- Chickweed
- Nettle

FOODS

- Dry fruits

LIFESTYLE

- Baking soda
- Lemon juice
- Coconut
- Apple-cider vinegar
- Aloe Vera
- Epsom salt
- Oatmeal

AVOID

- Caffeine
- Alcohol

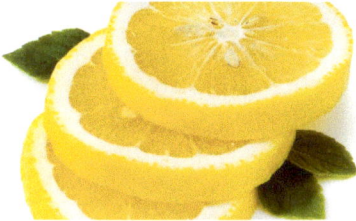

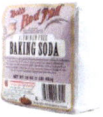

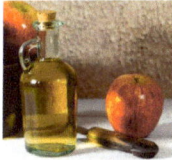

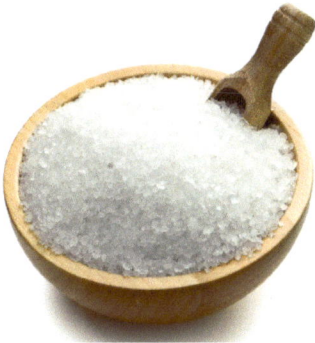

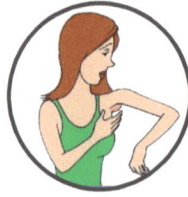

LYMPHOMA (NON-HODGKIN'S)

Non-Hodgkin's lymphoma is a cancer that develops in the B or T cells of your lymphatic system and spreads throughout your body. NHL also develops from white blood cells and indicates the person has nutritional deficiencies (due to genetic and lifestyle factors).

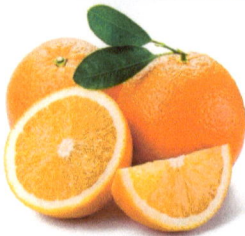

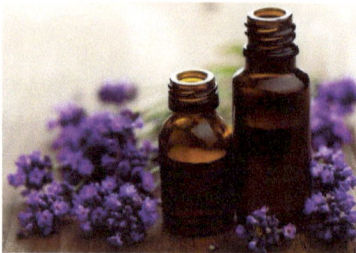

HOMEOPATHIC

- Chelidonium 6x take one every day for 3 weeks
- Galium 6c take one in the mornings.
- Hydrastis 6x take one every day
- Thuja 30c take 3x times a day
- Aparine 6c take one 4 times a day
- Ferrum Phos 30c take one a day
- Nux Vomica 30c take one a day
- Cadmium Sulph take one twice a day
- Ipecac 30c
- Chemotherapy mix 30c take when you are having chemotherapy to help with side affects.

ESSENTIAL OILS

- Lavender put 2 drops with 8 oz water and spray on your pillow
- Sandalwood put 2 drops in bath
- Orange put 2 drops in bath
- Ginger put 2 drops in a diffuser and
- Peppermint
- Sacred frankincense 2 drops mixed with 10 drops of carrier oil and rub under feet to help with side affects of chemotherapy

LYMPHOMA (NON-HODGKIN'S)
continued

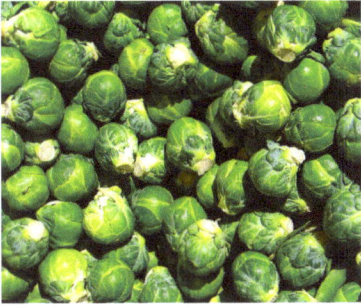

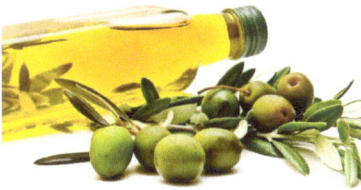

VITAMINS
Consult doctor before you take any vitamins

- Arginine
- Vitamin K
- Vitamin D
- EPA oils
- Ave power
- Shark oil
- Vitamin E400
- Essiac
- Amino acids
- Beta glucan
- Zinc
- Folic acid
- Melatonin
- Kava Kava
- Green tea peach
- Natural 401
- Natural 601
- Probiotic
- LifeOne
- Intestinal support
- Glutamine
- Activated charcoal if you have had chemotherapy it helps get rid of the toxins in your body but take it before you take any vitamins .

FOODS
- Organic salmon
- BPA-free sardines
- Olive oil
- Broccoli (raw or steamed)
- Cauliflower
- Brussels sprouts
- Leafy greens
- Red peppers
- Cucumber

LYMPHOMA (NON-HODGKIN'S)
continued

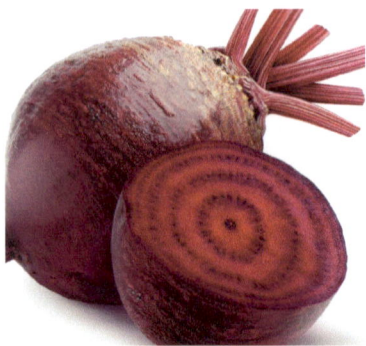

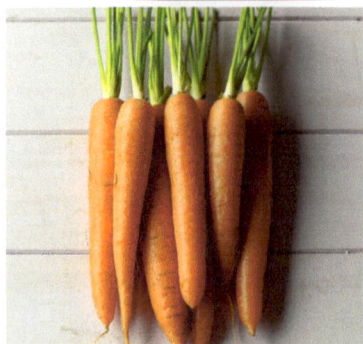

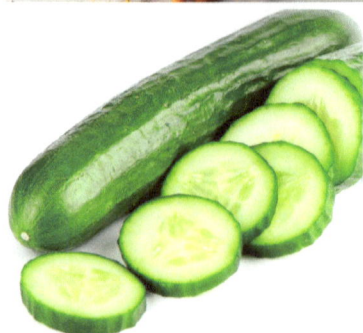

FOODS (CONTINUED)
- Bitter melon
- Daikon radish
- Beets
- Avocado
- Carrots
- Ginger
- Kale
- Chard
- Reishi mushroom
- Lemon
- Chai seed
- Flaxseeds
- Organic cottage cheese combined with flaxseed oil

LIFESTYLE
- Epsom salt in the bath
- Aluminium-free baking soda in the bath
- Lavender oil in the bath
- Infrared sauna
- Gentle massage for lymphatic drainage
- Reflexology
- Yoga
- Meditation
- Organic blackstrap molasses with aluminium-free baking soda
- Himalayan salt in baths or in water/foods
- Hydrotherapy
- Acupuncture
- Amino acid intravenously
- Organic apple-cider vinegar
- Immune colostrum protein shake
- Immune spray
- Silver colloidal
- Wheatgrass
- Green organic juices
- Body brushing
- Walking
- Breathing techniques

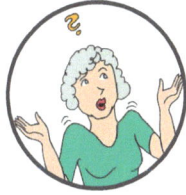

MEMORY

Forgetting where you left your keys and your jacket—this kind of memory problem can be helped by diet and by exercising the mind, e.g., doing crosswords.

HOMEOPATHIC
- Gelsemium 30c
- Lycopodium 30c

ESSENTIAL OILS
Inhaling 2 drops on a tissue with carrier oil
- Rosemary
- Lemon

VITAMINS
Take one a day with food.
- Omega-3, -6, and -9
- Vitamin C
- Magnesium

FOODS
- Salmon
- Mackerel
- Sardines
- Rainbow fish
- Trout
- Tuna
- Avocados
- Bananas
- Apples
- Eggs

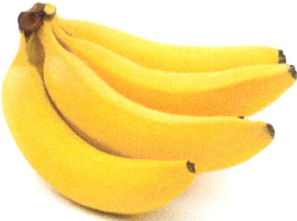

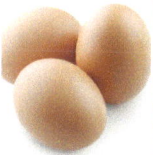

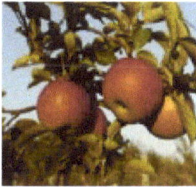

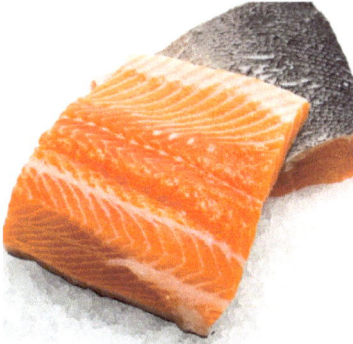

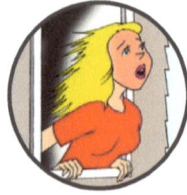

MENOPAUSE

Menopause is the cessation of the functioning of a woman's reproductive system, which usually happens around age fifty, although it may occur before or after this age. It signals the transition from the reproductive phase to the nonreproductive phase in a woman's life. The most common symptoms related to menopause include hot flashes, menstrual irregularity, depressive mood and irritability, loss of libido, and vaginal dryness.

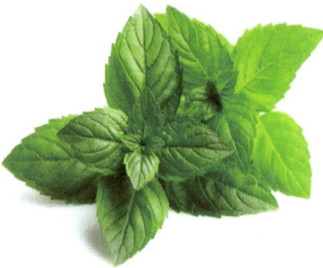

HOMEOPATHIC
One dose at fifteen minutes intervals for 3-4 doses

- Lachesis 30c
- Sepia 30c
- Folliculinum 6c
- Pulsatilla 30c
- Magnesium Phosphate 30c

ESSENTIAL OILS
In the bath or inhale 1 to 2 drops

- Clary sage
- Anise
- Fennel
- Lavender
- Coriander
- Sage
- Rose
- Lemon
- Peppermint

VITAMINS
- Calcium
- Vitamin B
- Vitamin D
- Vitamin E
- Vitamin K
- Magnesium
- Estroven natural tablets
- Immune system IP6
- Essiac
- Shark-liver oil
- Alpha lipoic acid

MENOPAUSE
continued

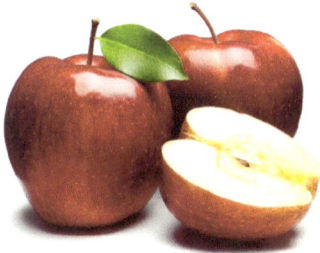

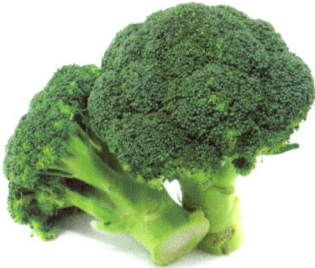

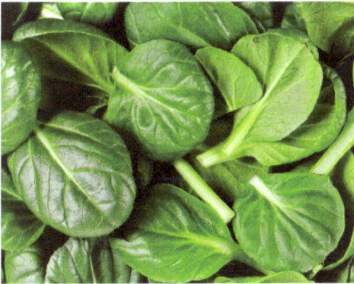

VITAMINS (CONTINUED)
- Andrographis
- Amino acids
- Zinc
- Beta glucan

FOODS
- Sardines
- Organic salmon
- Broccoli
- Flaxseeds
- Quinoa
- Barley
- Lentils
- Apples
- Spinach
- Olive oil
- Organic red wine
- Yam
- Mixed vegetables
- Sheep yogurt
- Goat yogurt
- Coconut yogurt
- Cucumbers

HERBS
- Vitex berry
- Ashwagandha
- Black cohosh
- Milk thistle (helps clean the liver)
- Geranium (helps to balance your hormones)
- Clary sage (if you suffer from nervous tension)
- Cardamom
- Peppermint
- Sweet fennel
- Dong Quai

MENOPAUSE
continued

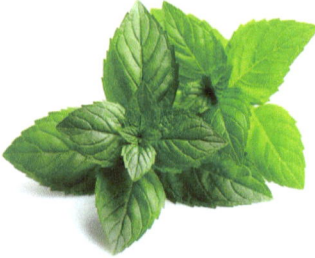

HERBS (CONTINUED)
- Chasteberry
- Ginger
- Valerian
- Cramp bark
- Evening primrose
- Yam cream

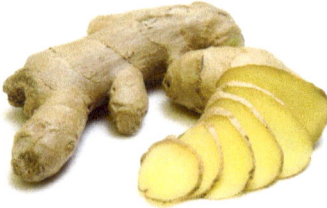

LIFESTYLE
- Emerita (cream)
- Yoga
- Acupuncture
- Sunbathing (Vitamin D)
- Breathing techniques

AVOID
- Refined sugar
- Caffeine
- Spicy foods
- Salt

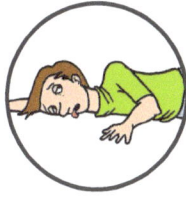

MENTAL EXHAUSTION

Mental exhaustion is becoming one of the more prevalent problems today. Symptoms of mental exhaustion include feeling constantly tired and being unable to concentrate.

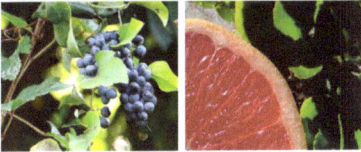

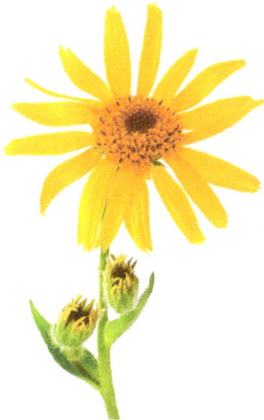

HOMEOPATHIC
One dose 2-3 times a day reduce with improvement

- Lycopodium
- Nux Vomica
- Picric Acid
- Arnica Montana
- Kali Phosphoricum
- Phosphoric Acid
- Silica
- Cocculus

FOODS THAT HELP
- Grapefruit

LIFESTYLE
Take one a day with your doctors recommendation

- 5-HTP supplement
- L-Theanine
- B-complex
- Omega-3, -6, and -9

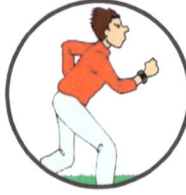

METABOLIC SYNDROME

Metabolic syndrome is a disorder of energy storage and is often associated with obesity, and elevated blood pressure causing an increased risk of developing cardiovascular disease and diabetes.

HOMEOPATHIC
Take one a day

- Carbo Vegetabillis 30c
- Phosphorous 30c
- Arsenicum Album 30c
- Calcarea-Carbonica 30c
- Rhus Toxicodendron 30c
- Crataegus 30c
- Aconite 30c
- Electritas 30c

ESSENTIAL OILS
8 drops in the bath.

- Lemon
- Tangerine
- Grapefruit
- Bergamot
- Ocotea

VITAMINS
After meals

- Vitamin B complex
- Vitamin D
- L-Carnitine
- Coenzyme

FOODS

- Walnuts
- Asparagus
- Beans
- Cruciferous vegetables
- Celery
- Cucumbers

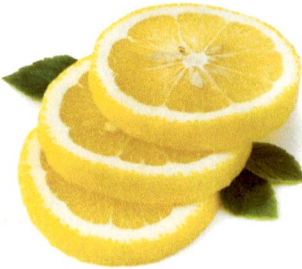
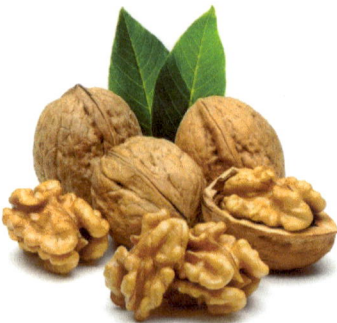

METABOLIC SYNDROME
continued

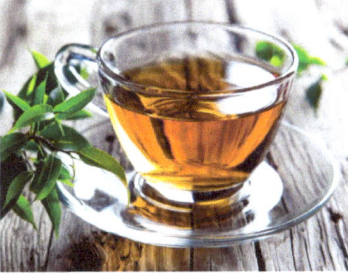

HERBAL TEAS
Drink up to 3-4 cups a day.

- White oolong
- Green
- Porangaba
- Peppermint
- White
- Rose
- Feiyan

AVOID

- Alcohol
- Refined sugars

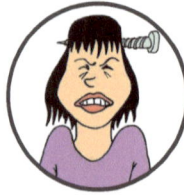

MIGRAINE

Migraines occur most often in women due to fluctuations in the level of the hormone estrogen. As a result, women tend to suffer from migraines around the time of menstruation, when estrogen levels are lowest. Men are also susceptible to migraines.

HOMEOPATHIC
One dose every 15-30 minutes

- Bryonia 30c
- Nat Mur 30c
- Iris Ver 30c
- Nux Vomica 30c

VITAMINS
after meals

- Vitamin C

LIFESTYLE

- Primrose oil
- Rutin
- Garlic

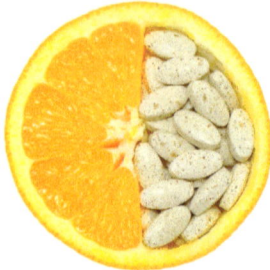

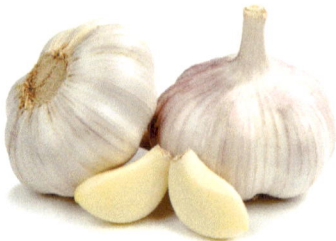

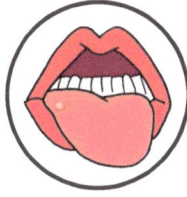

MOUTH ULCER

A mouth ulcer is an ulcer that occurs on the mucous membrane of the mouth. Mouth ulcers are common, usually occurring in conjunction with other diseases and by many different mechanisms. Although mouth ulcers can be uncomfortable and painful, they are not usually serious.

HOMEOPATHIC
One dose three times a day reducing with improvements
- Nitric Acid 30c
- Mercurius Solublis 30c
- Borax venata 30c

ESSENTIAL OILS
2 drops of each in a 10 oz cup and swish around the mouth before spitting it out
- Peppermint oil
- Tea tree

FOODS
- Basil
- Onion
- Coconut milk
- Orange juice

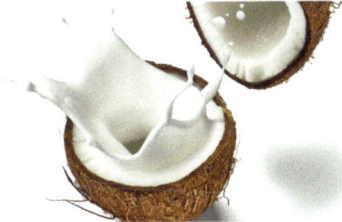

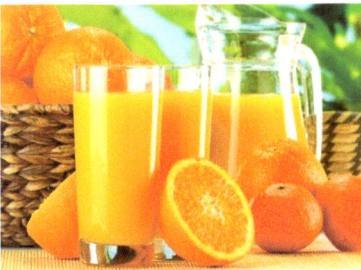

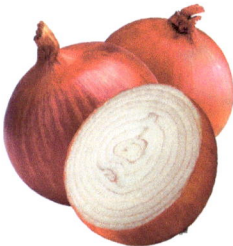

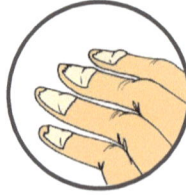

NAILS

Nails are made of protein, and depending on your genes, they can become brittle with age. Nail fungus may cause your nails to discolor, thicken, and crumble at the edge. Nail fungus is called onychomycosis and tinea unguium.

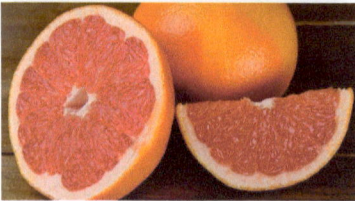

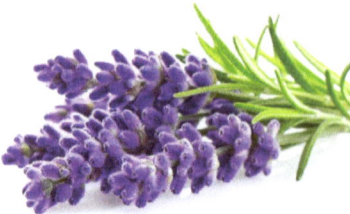

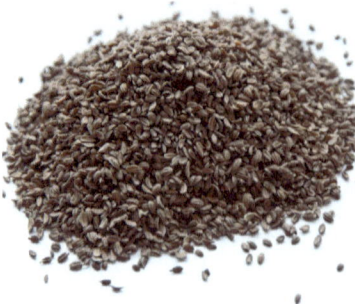

HOMEOPATHIC
One dose morning and one in evening

- Silicea 6c
- Graphites naturalis 6c
- Fluoric Acid 6c

ESSENTIAL OILS
Soak nails in oil for 5 mins.

- Myrrh
- Lavender
- Carrot seed
- Grapefruit
- Rosemary
- Roman chamomile

VITAMINS
Take after meals

- Biotin
- Zinc
- Calcium
- Magnesium
- Bio seal

LIFESTYLE
Take up to 10 drops in the morning after meals

- Herb silicea
- Horsetail tea
- Lemon and oil

AVOID
- Cutting cuticles since they act as a barrier to bacteria

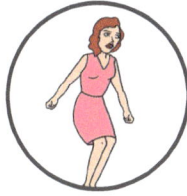

PREMENSTRUAL TENSION

PMT is a condition that occurs before and during a woman's menstrual cycle. PMT has a multitude of physical and psychological complaints and is extremely variable from one person to another, with symptoms ranging from mild to incapacitating. It is likely that three out of four women get some degree of PMT, and approximately one-third suffer sufficiently to seek medical help.

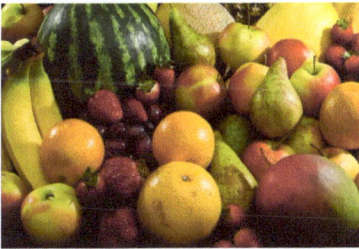

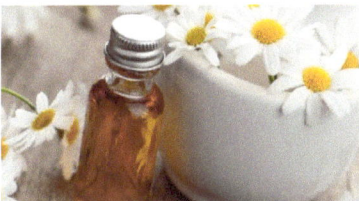

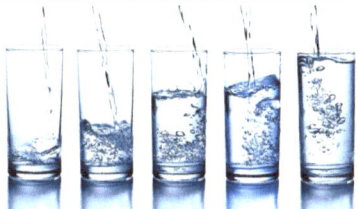

HOMEOPATHIC
One dose morning and one in evening starting on day twelve of the cycle.

- Sepia Succus 30c
- Lachesis 30c
- Pulsatilla 30c

ESSENTIAL OILS
2 drops of oil with 10ml carrier oil. Massage in.

- Geranium
- Rose
- Bergamot
- Jasmine
- Neroli
- Lavender
- Camomile

FOODS
- Mixed seeds (pumpkin, sunflower, and sesame)
- Fruit
- Vegetables
- Berries
- Foods rich in potassium (tomatoes, peanuts, potatoes, bananas, peaches, figs, and dates)
- Muesli and nuts
- Eggs
- Protein shakes
- Increase fiber in your diet

LIFESTYLE
- Calcium
- Herbs such as agnus castus, black cohosh, and dong quai take 10 drops in 8oz water

79

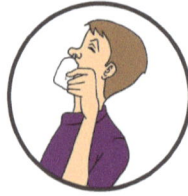

SINUSITIS

Acute sinusitis (acute rhinosinusitis) causes the cavities around your nasal passages (sinuses) to become inflamed and swollen. This interferes with drainage and causes mucus to build up. Sinusitis is most often caused by the common cold. Other triggers include bacteria, allergies, and fungal infections.

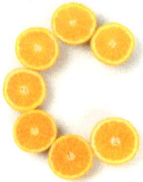

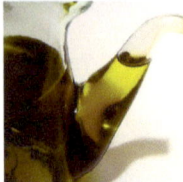

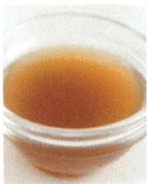

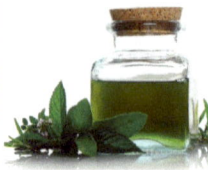

HOMEOPATHIC
One dose 4 times a day
- Kali-Bichromicum 6c
- Thuja occidentalis 6c

ESSENTIAL OILS
3 drops of eucalyptus, peppermint and rosemary with 20 ml of carrier oil. Massage the neck, chest, hands and sole of the feet.
- Peppermint (inhaled)
- Rosemary (inhaled)
- Eucalyptus (inhaled)
- Oregano (inhaled)

FOODS
- Apple-cider vinegar one tspn in 8 oz of water
- Turmeric compound known as curcumin one a day

LIFESTYLE
- Vitamin C one a day

AVOID
- Dairy

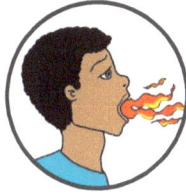

SORE THROAT

Sore throats are commonly caused by a virus. Fungal infections can also cause a sore throat, usually in people with weakened immune systems.

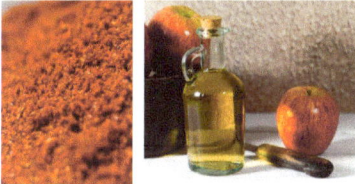

HOMEOPATHIC

One dose every two to three hours and reduce with improvements

- Mercurius solublis 6c
- Belladonna 6c
- Lachesis 30c
- Aconite 30c

FOODS

- Slippery elm
- Licorice root
- Honeysuckle
- Lemon
- Organic Apple Cider Vinegar one tspn in 6oz water and drink twice a day
- Cayenne
- Honey
- Sage

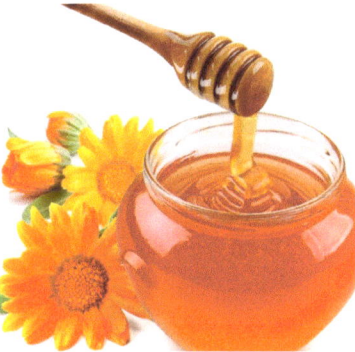

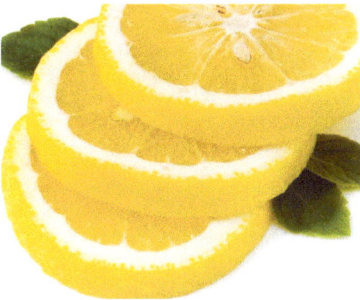

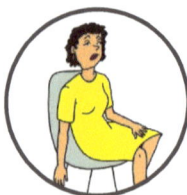

STROKE

A stroke occurs when the blood supply to part of your brain is interrupted or severely reduced, depriving brain tissue of oxygen and food. Within minutes, brain cells begin to die. Most strokes have a sudden or rapidly evolving onset.

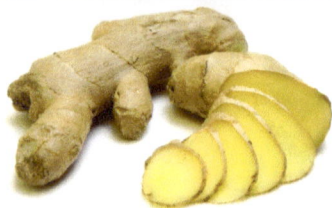

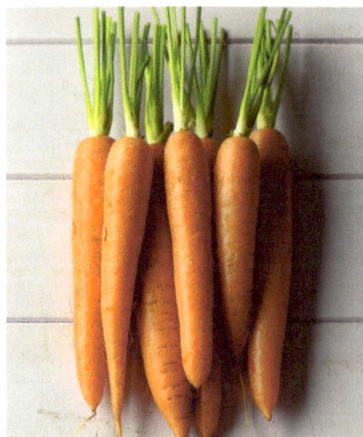

HOMEOPATHIC
One dose morning and one in evening

- Aconite 30c
- Arnica 30c

ESSENTIAL OILS
In bath

- Lavender
- Peppermint
- Rosemary

FOODS

- Ginger
- Turmeric
- Carrot
- Spinach
- Pineapple
- Astragalus
- Vegetable juice
- Fish oils

HERBAL TEAS
Drink up to 3 cups a day.

- Green
- Horsetail

HERBS

- Kava kava take twice a day
- Hawthorn take 10 drops in 8 oz of water for a month

STROKE
continued

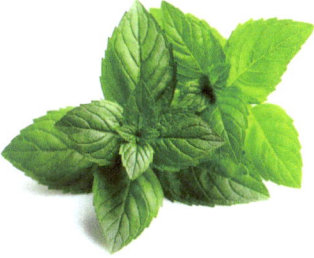

LIFESTYLE
Take one a day with meals
- Ginkgo biloba – improves circulation
- B6/B12 folic acid

AVOID
- Too much meat
- Dairy products
- Fatty foods

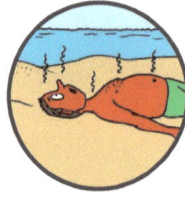

SUNBURN

Mild sunburn can cause redness, pain, and slight swelling for about three to seven days. Skin may peel and itch.

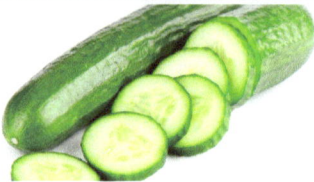

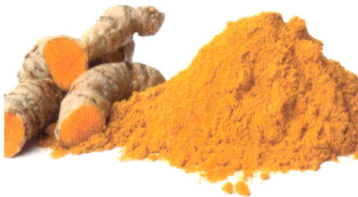

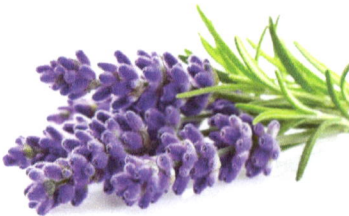

HOMEOPATHIC
One dose every two hours until relief
- Aconite 30c
- Cantharis 30c
- Sol 30c

ESSENTIAL OILS
10 oz filtered water and 2-4 drops of lavender placed in a dark glass bottle. Spray where needed.
- Lavender
- Coconut

FOODS
- Yogurt
- Turmeric and plain yogurt apply on the skin
- Aloe vera gel apply to the skin
- Cucumber placed on the skin cools it down.
- Mayonnaise placed on the skin helps calm burns.

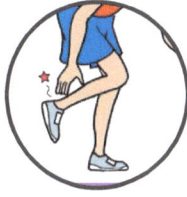

TENDINITIS

Tendinitis is an inflammation of a tendon, the thick cord that attaches bone to muscle, usually caused by a physical trauma.

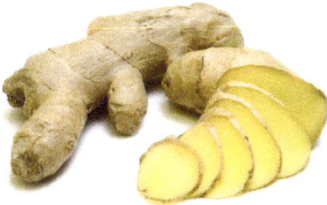

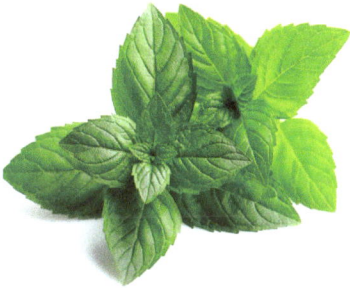

HOMEOPATHIC

One dose every 2-4 times a day

- Meadow sweet 6c
- Magnesia-Phos 6c
- Bryonia 6c
- Berberis 6c
- Traumeel gel apply on the area

ESSENTIAL OILS

2 drops of each oil in the bath.

- Lemongrass
- Peppermint

HERBS

- Ginger one a day with food
- Turmeric one a day with food.
- Bromelain one a day with food.
- White willow one a day with food.
- Fenugreek one a day with food.

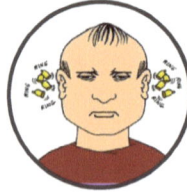

TINNITUS

Tinnitus is associated with decreased hearing. Allergies, tumors, and problems in the heart and blood vessels, jaws, and neck can cause tinnitus. High blood cholesterol clogs arteries that supply oxygen to the nerves of the inner ear. Advancing age is generally accompanied by a certain amount of hearing nerve impairment and tinnitus.

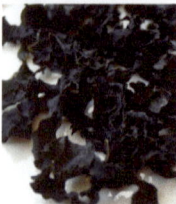

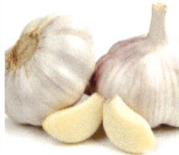

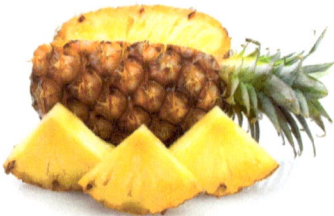

HOMEOPATHIC

One dose at intervals of thirty minutes for 3-4 doses. Reduce dosage with improvement.

- Carbo Vegetabilis 6c
- Causticum 6c
- Chininum-Sulphuricum 6c

FOODS

- Fresh pineapples
- Garlic
- Kelp

LIFESTYLE

- Coenzyme Q10 one a day
- Bayberry bark
- Hawthorn leaf one a day
- Juniper
- Ginkgo one a day with food
- Zinc one a day with food
- Cranio-sacral therapy

AVOID

- Excessive salt
- Caffeine
- Alcohol
- MSG
- Cheese
- Chocolate
- High-fat foods

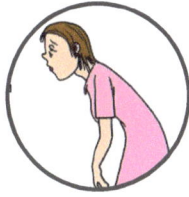

THYROID (UNDERACTIVE)

The thyroid gland, which controls the metabolic rate and is part of the endocrine system that produces hormones, is found below the voice box. Hypothyroidism, or underactive thyroid, develops when the thyroid gland fails to produce or secrete as much thyroxine (T4) as the body needs.

HOMEOPATHIC
One a day

- Thyroidinum 30c

ESSENTIAL OILS
One drop in the bath

- Peppermint
- Clove
- Spearmint

FOODS

- Kelp
- Chicken
- Beef
- Parsley
- Bananas
- Iodine
- Coconut oil

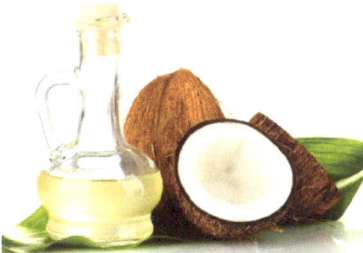

HERBAL TEAS
Drink 2-3 cups a day

- Black walnut
- Irish moss

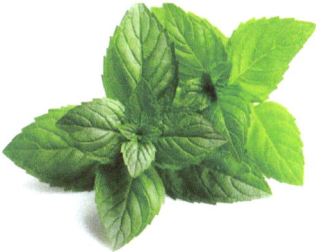

LIFESTYLE

- Exercise

AVOID

- Foods that contain white flour (e.g., white bread)
- Foods that are high in saturated fats

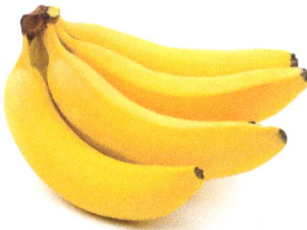

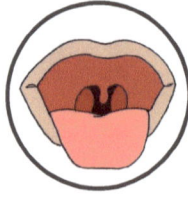

TONSILLITIS

Tonsillitis or inflammation of the tonsils is a painful condition of the throat that can also cause high temperatures.

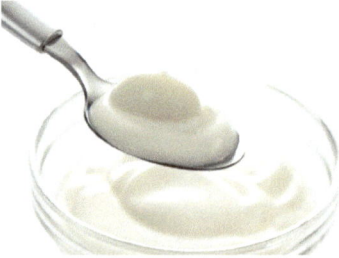

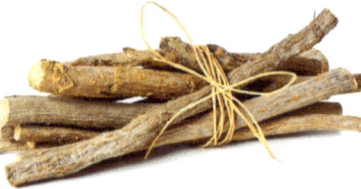

HOMEOPATHIC

One dose every two to three hours and reduce with improvements.

- Aconite 30c
- Belladonna 30c
- Baryta Carb 30c

ESSENTIAL OILS

2 drops in the bath.

- Eucalyptus
- Peppermint

FOODS

- Liquids to keep hydrated
- Soft foods, e.g., yogurts and winter squash
- Licorice root 10 drops in 8 oz of filter water

AVOID

- Acidic drinks like grapefruit juice and lemonade
- Caffeine

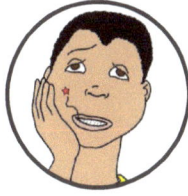

TOOTHACHE

Toothache is pain in the teeth and/or gums/jaw caused by disease. A toothache can be caused by a problem that does not originate from a tooth or the jaw.

HOMEOPATHIC
One dose every hour. Reduce with improvement.

- Aconite 6c
- Belladonna 6c
- Chamomilla 6c

VITAMINS
As directed

- Vitamin C

FOODS

- Ginger
- Garlic
- Sea salt
- Sesame seeds

LIFESTYLE

- Echinacea

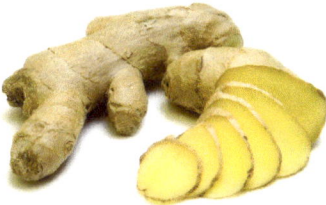

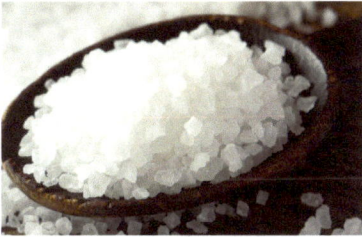

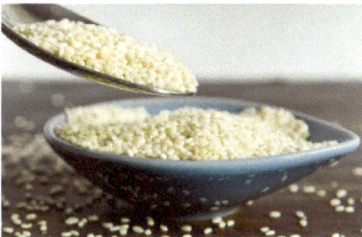

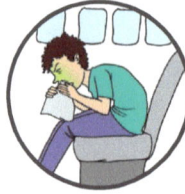

TRAVEL SICKNESS

Motion sickness (also known as travel sickness) is characterized by an uncomfortable, queasy sensation experienced when traveling by car, train, airplane, and boat, or by using a playground swing or riding some amusement–park rides.

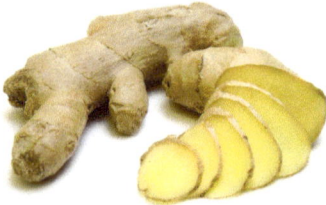

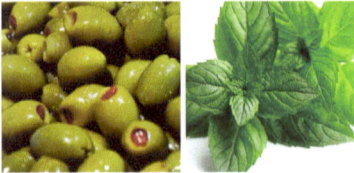

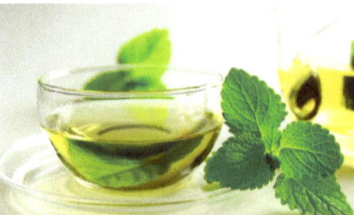

HOMEOPATHIC
3 doses a day

- Argentum Nitricum 6c
- Borax 6c
- Cocculus Indicus 6c
- Kali Bichromicum 6c
- Nux Vomica 6c

ESSENTIAL OILS
1 drop in bath

- Ginger
- Nutmeg
- Peppermint

FOODS

- Olives
- Fresh ginger
- Fresh mint tea
- Ginger ale

AVOID

- Spicy foods
- Alcohol

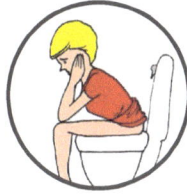

URINARY RETENTION

Urinary retention occurs when the bladder does not empty completely.

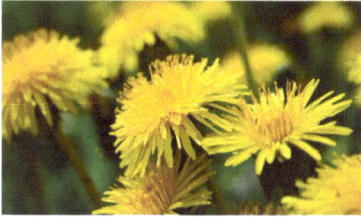

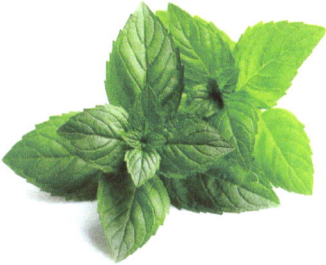

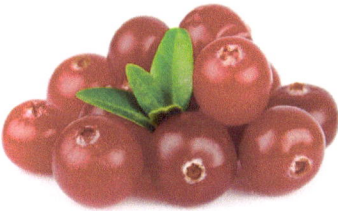

HOMEOPATHIC

One dose 4-5 times a day. Reduce with improvement.

- Aconite 6c
- Digitalis 30c
- Apis mellifica 30c

ESSENTIAL OILS

Put 3 drops in the bath

- Peppermint

FOODS

- Dandelion
- India licorice
- Cranberry
- Uva ursi leaf 1 a day
- Pineapples
- Baking soda take half a spoon in 5 oz water

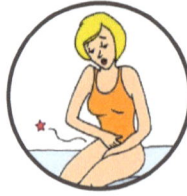

URINARY TRACT INFECTION

Urinary tract infections are caused by microbes, such as bacteria, that overcome the body's defenses in the urinary tract. The majority of urinary tract infections are caused by the E.coli bacterium.

The most common UTIs occur mainly in women and affect the urethra and bladder. Cystitis is the most common type of urinary tract infection. UTIs can affect cognitive functions in extreme cases.

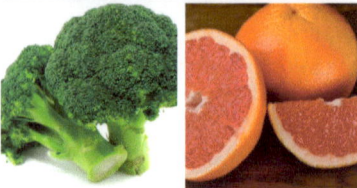

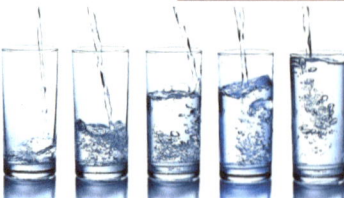

HOMEOPATHIC

- Aconite 30c
- Apis 6c
- Berberis 30c
- Cantharis 30c
- Sepia 6c
- Staph 6c

ESSENTIAL OILS

Mix 2 drops of lavender, eucalyptus and tea tree

- Lavender
- Bergamot
- Cajeput
- Eucalyptus
- Tea tree
- Sage

VITAMINS

Take one a day after meals

- Vitamin C take one a day with food
- Cranberry capsule one a day
- D-Mannose powder one tspn in 8oz water
- Jarro-Dophilusone a day
- Probiotic take one before breakfast

FOODS

- Plenty of water
- Cranberries
- Blueberries
- Broccoli
- Cauliflower
- Grapefruit
- Parsley

URINARY TRACT INFECTION
continued

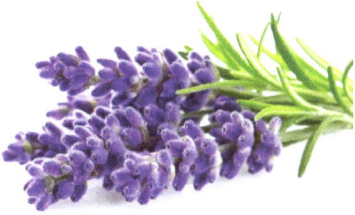

FOODS (CONTINUED)

- Aluminium -free baking soda
- Kefir yogurts
- Fermented products

AVOID

- Coffee
- Alcohol
- Spicy foods
- Nicotine
- Carbonated water

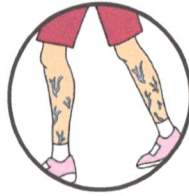

VARICOSE VEINS

Varicose veins are enlarged veins with a knotted look that are caused by poor circulation. The areas most commonly affected are the legs and feet.

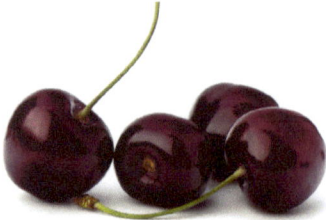

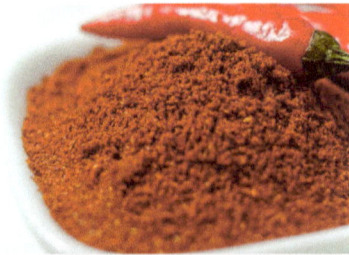

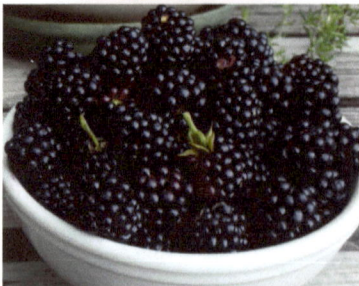

HOMEOPATHIC

- Arnica Montana 30c
- Cal-carb 30c
- Carbo Vegetabilis 30c
- Hamamelis 30c

ESSENTIAL OILS

- Cypress
- Rosemary
- Lemon
- Bergamot

FOODS

- Apple-cider vinegar
- Dried basil
- Cherries
- Blackberries
- Pineapple
- Cayenne pepper
- Fresh ginger
- Natto

LIFESTYLE

- Walking (to help increase circulation)

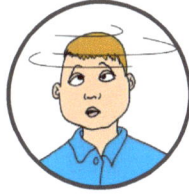

VERTIGO

Vertigo is a disease associated with the posterior semicircular canals of the inner ear that causes an abnormal sensation of the surrounding environment, such as continuously spinning, whirling, or moving. As a result, a vertigo patient suffers loss of balance.

HOMEOPATHIC

- Cocculus indicus 30c
- Lobelia inflata 30c
- Gelsemium 30c

ESSENTIAL OILS

- Lavender
- Peppermint
- Neroli
- Anise

FOODS

- Celery
- Basil
- Pine nuts

LIFESTYLE

- Ginkgo biloba
- Valerian

AVOID

- Fatty foods
- Eggs
- Dairy

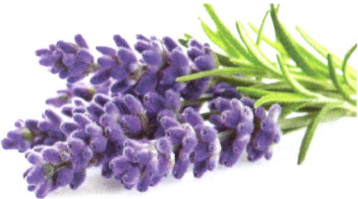

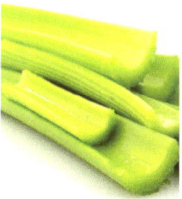

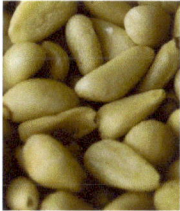

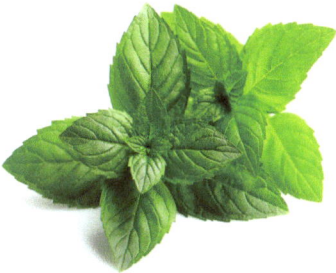

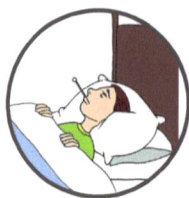

VIRAL INFECTION

A viral infection can lower the immune system and allow in different illnesses, such as colds, headaches, flu, and sore throat with a fever.

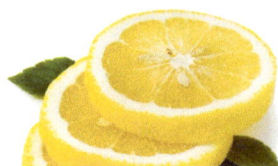

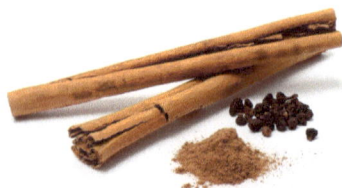

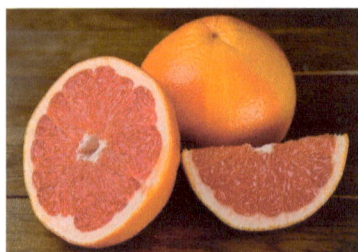

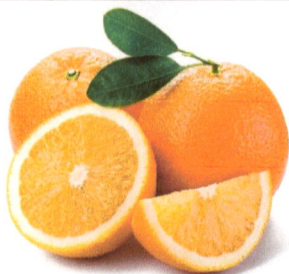

HOMEOPATHIC
One dose every 30 minutes
- Aconitum 30c
- Belladonna 6c
- Gelsemium 30c

VITAMINS
- Vitamin B
- Vitamin C

ESSENTIAL OILS
Rub feet with 2 drops
- Eucalyptus
- Clove
- Lemon
- Rosemary
- Cinnamon

FOODS
- Grapefruit
- Oranges

AVOID
- Refined sugars
- Carbohydrates (e.g. potatoes, bread)

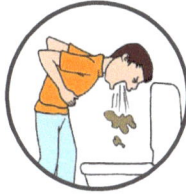

VOMITING

Vomiting is the act of throwing up unwanted food and drink from the stomach. Vomiting and nausea are both usually caused by a viral gastroenteritis, excessive acidity in the body, or dehydration. Vomiting can also be the side effect of medication.

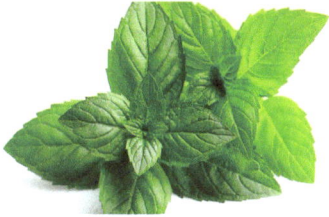

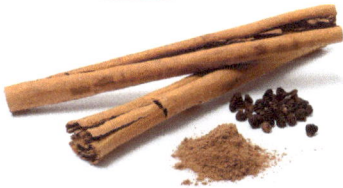

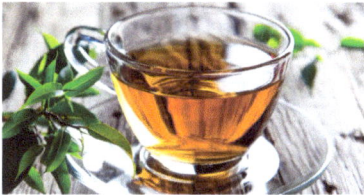

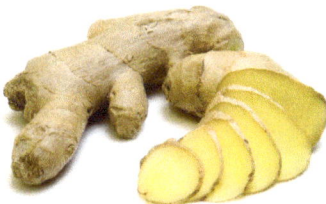

HOMEOPATHIC

One dose every 2-4 hours

- Arsenicum Album 30c
- Nux Vomica 30c
- Colocynthis 30c

ESSENTIAL OILS

Mix 2 drops of each and mix with carrier oil and apply behind ears

- Peppermint
- Ginger

FOODS

- Foods easy to digest such as yogurt, bananas, white rice, or cottage cheese
- Diluted juice, vegetable broth, or rice water
- Lime juice in water
- Cinnamon
- Cloves
- Apple juice
- Digestion enzymes
- Papaya

HERBAL TEAS

drink up to three to four cups a day

- Ginger
- Mint

AVOID

- Heavy, rich foods
- Sweets

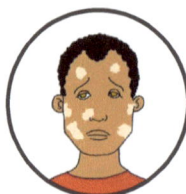

VITILIGO

Vitiligo is the loss of pigmentation or patches of de-pigmented skin. Vitiligo is an autoimmune condition in which the body attacks its own pigment cells.

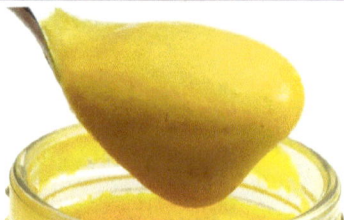

HOMEOPATHIC
Take one three times a day

- Nat Carbonicum 30c
- Sulphur 30c
- Silica 30c

VITAMINS
Take one a day with food

- Ginkgo
- Folic acid
- Vitamin B12

ESSENTIAL OILS
Use 2 drops mixed in with carrier oil and apply where you have vitiligo.

- Turmeric
- Mustard
- Ginger
- Lavender
- Tea tree

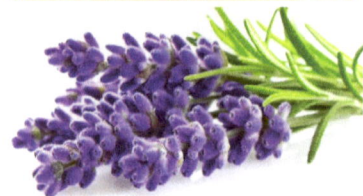

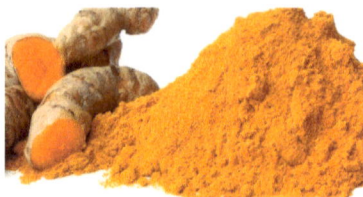

HERBAL TEAS
Drink up to 3 to 4 cups a day.

- Green
- Oregano

FOODS

- Black pepper
- Olive oil
- Ginger
- Garlic
- Turmeric

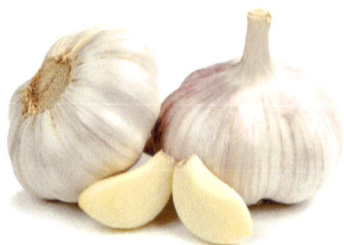

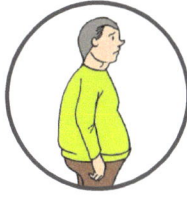

WATER RETENTION

Water retention (also known as fluid retention) is the accumulation of fluid in the circulatory system or within the tissues or cavities of the body. Water retention occurs when water leaks from the blood into the body tissues.

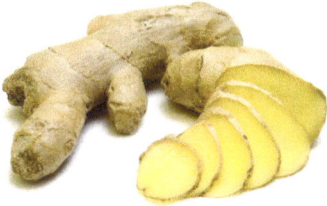

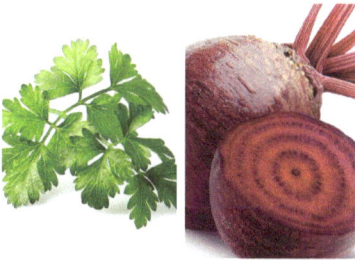

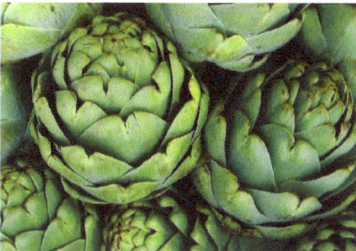

HOMEOPATHIC
One dose 2-4 hours
- Apis Mellifica
- Cal Carb

ESSENTIAL OILS
Mix two drops of lemon and 2 drops of Geranium in the bath.
- Geranium
- Lemon
- Juniper
- Cypress

FOODS
- Parsley
- Beetroot
- Artichoke
- Ginger

HERBS
Take up to 10 drops in 8 oz of water
- Uva Ursi
- Horse chestnut
- Buchu

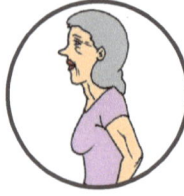

WRINKLES

Wrinkles are a sign of aging but can also be caused by sun exposure. As the body gets older, the skin texture changes, getting thinner and losing elasticity.

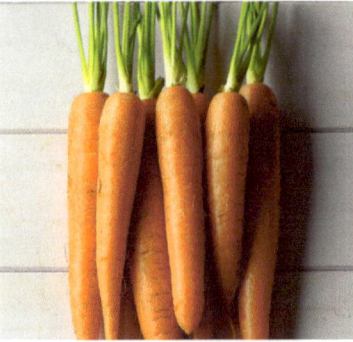

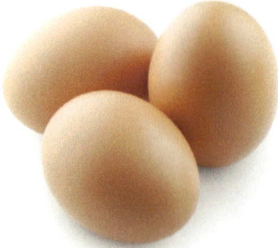

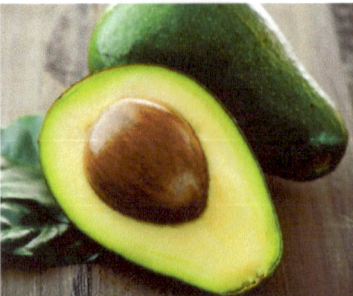

HOMEOPATHIC
One dose morning and one in evening

- Silica 6c
- Nat Mur 6c
- Kali Mur 6c
- Sulphur 6c

ESSENTIAL OILS
Mix two drops in carrier oil and massage very gently on face.

- Sandalwood
- Myrrh
- Neroli
- Clary sage
- Geranium
- Emu
- Rosewood
- Frankincense
- Patchouli

FOODS

- Avocado
- Salmon
- Buckwheat
- Blueberries
- Brazil nuts
- Carrots
- Eggs

HERBAL TEAS
drink up to 3 to 4 cups a day

- White
- Green

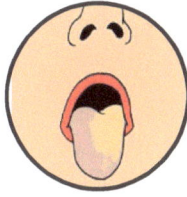

YEAST INFECTIONS

Vaginal infections are infections or inflammation of the vagina. Yeast infections are caused by fungal candida. This fungus is associated with intense itching, swelling, and irritation.

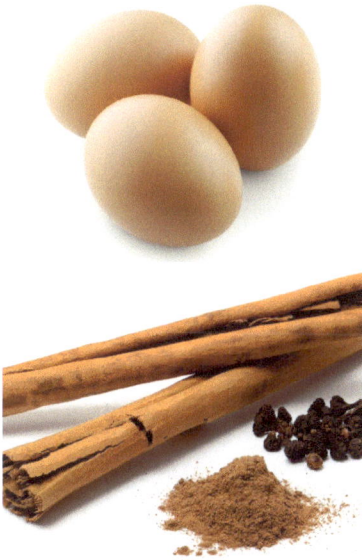

HOMEOPATHIC
One dose morning and one in evening
- Cal-carb 30c
- Nat-Mur 30c
- Borax 30c

ESSENTIAL OILS
2-3 drops of each in the bath
- Oregano
- Tea tree
- Cinnamon

VITAMINS
- Probiotics take one on a empty stomach
- Vitamin C one a aday with meals
- Zinc one a day with meals
- Beta carotene one a day with meals

FOODS
- Organic apple-cider vinegar take one tspn in 5 oz of water twice a day
- Egg whites

HERBS
- Pau'arco
- Calendula
- Grapefruit-seeds extract
- Golden seal

YEAST INFECTIONS
continued

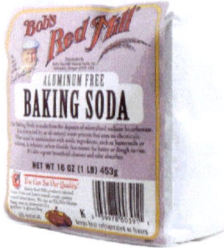

LIFESTYLE

- Wearing loose clothes
- Meditation
- Boric-acid suppositories
- Good night's sleep
- Epsom salts
- Baking soda containing aluminum

AVOID

- Sugars
- Refined foods
- Tight pants
- Deodorants

ABOUT THE AUTHOR, OUSSHA SHLAIMOUN

I recall being drawn to nature from an early age. I grew up in a very modest neighborhood in London, England, in the 1970s, a place where we learned not to expect too much from life. Mum and Dad spent all hours working to keep a roof over our heads and food on the table, leaving my younger sister and I home alone most of the day. Left to our own devices, we learned to keep ourselves busy around our small one-bedroom apartment.

Whilst friends played in the street or watched television, I was busy cooking, cleaning, and washing/ironing clothes. Thinking back now, we had a tough childhood, but at the time it didn't seem so bad. I guess when you don't know any better, you just get on with it. My only escape was when I would go into our small garden where I would grow and cultivate plants. In the garden, I didn't feel inferior (even if it was only a temporary escape). In fact, gardening was empowering. I could grow flowers, pick petals, and produce all types of concoctions. Writing this reminds me of the sweet, soft smell of rose water I would make from crushed rose petals or the soaps and oils I would make from the lavender I had grown. I think I must have my mum's genes; she was always making natural potions to help sooth us when we were sick. I remember watching her and wanting to be just like her.

I was a sickly child, always suffering from one complaint or another. My Achilles' heel was my stomach, and boy did I suffer from it. Growing up in England in the '70s, we were forced to drink cow's milk at school. Most kids loved it, but I hated it. I would rather go hungry than drink milk, but we didn't have a choice back then. I can't recall how many doctors I saw growing up, but I do recall that they all prescribed antibiotics—that was the norm those days. It would take some forty years before I would realize the cause of my complaint: I had an intolerance to milk. But by the time I realized the issue, the damage was done. Our bodies talk to us and tell us what is good for us and what isn't; we just need to learn to listen.

The irony is that as I grew older and began to work, I could afford to eat the foods I could have only dreamt of as a child, but I was unable to because I had developed an intolerance to almost everything I ate, an intolerance possibly caused by the massive amounts of antibiotics I had been prescribed as a child. Once again, I consulted numerous physicians who almost always put me on a diet fit for a small rabbit. It was obvious no one could help, so that's when I decided to take my health into my own hands and realized I needed to turn to nature for an answer.

I enrolled into university and studied a degree in homeopathy at The College for Homeopathic Education in Regents College, a campus of The Middlesex University. But after I finished that course, I didn't stop there; I read and I read. My thirst for knowledge had been ignited, and I became an information junky. I read articles and research papers on all types of ailments and remedies. At the time I didn't realize how life-changing it was or how much it would help me and my family.

More recently, I finished a one-year intensive course in integrative nutrition because I believe it is important we understand what it is we are eating to fuel the fire within us.

❘ CONNECT WITH OUSSHA

Website: http://rightberry.com/

Email: oussha@rightberry.com

❘ IN GRATITUDE TO YOU...

I would be so grateful if you could take a minute or two to share what you loved about this book and provide an honest review on our Amazon sales page.

- Oussha

www.ingramcontent.com/pod-product-compliance
Lightning Source LLC
Chambersburg PA
CBHW040127270326
41927CB00001B/13